D0880986

E. A. Stead, Jr.
What This Patient Needs Is a Doctor

E. A. Stead, Jr.

What This Patient Needs Is a Doctor

Edited by:
Galen S. Wagner
Bess Cebe
Marvin P. Rozear

Carolina Academic Press
Durham, North Carolina

Grateful acknowledgement is made to the following publishers for permission to repro-
duce excerpts from the following publications: *Just Say For Me* (World Press Inc.),
Medical Times, Journal of Medical Education, New England Journal of Medicine, Pharos
of AOA, Annals of Internal Medicine, Archives of Internal Medicine, Journal of American
Medical Association, Disease-a-Month, *The Future of Medical Education* (Duke Press),
Modern Medicine, *Signs and Symptoms* (J. P. Lippincott), *Principles of Internal Medicine*
(McGraw-Hill), Journal of Clinical Investigation, and American Journal of Diseases of
Children.

Carolina Academic Press
P. O. Box 8791
Durham, N.C. 27707

FOREWORD

"If I may use a figure, [Nature] has established the general intellectual level of the race at say, six feet. Take any billion men and stand them in a mass, and their headtops will make a floor—a floor as level as a table. That floor represents the intellectual altitude of the masses—and it never changes. Here and there, miles apart, a head will project above it a matter of one intellectual inch, so to speak—men of mark in science, law, war, commerce, etc.; in a spread of 5,000 miles you will find three heads that project still an inch higher, men of national fame—and one that is higher than those by two inches, maybe three—a man of (temporarily) world-renown; and finally, somewhere around the circumference of the globe, you will find once in five centuries of waiting, one majestic head which overtops the highest of all the others. . . . Now in that view you have the ordinary man of all nations; you have the here-and-there man that is larger-brained and becomes distinguished; you have the still rarer man of still wider and more lasting distinction; and in that final head rising solitary out of the stretch of the ages, you have the limit of Nature's output.

From Mark Twain, *Letters From the Earth*

"People respect, admire and love Dr. Stead because within the turmoil of his life he seems to have a simplicity, directness and detachment which makes him able to be calm and helpful. Furthermore, his character is virtuous. In times when most men are so selfish, his qualities of selflessness and dedication loom large.

"When speaking with him, I was struck with his existential state. He seemed to be deeply concentrated within himself and able to be fully in the moment. As we spoke about the nature of human suffering, he pointed out that most people live their lives in the past, or in the future, both of which don't actually exist at the moment. He shared his experience that if one is totally and selflessly aware of the present, life is magnificent. He experienced a continual 'flow of exciting, meaningful moment'. He felt that suffering is due to people's preoccupation with the past or the future without attention to the moment. He felt that human beings have a deep rational capacity for reason, clarity, virtue and love; but that we are rarely aware of it."

John Horton, M.D.
Duke Alumni Register; Vol. 60, October 1974

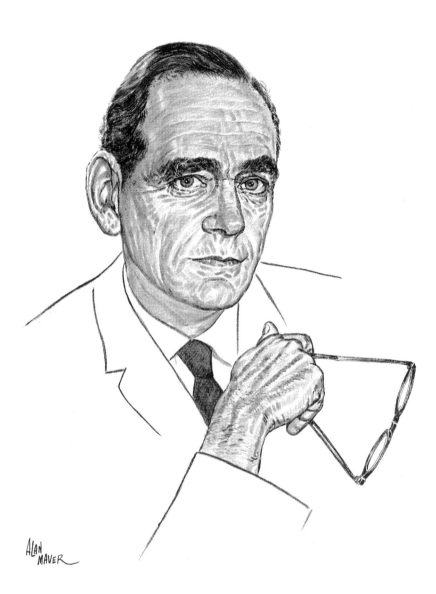

PREFACE

The idea for this book originated in discussions in the summer of 1976 between two of us (GSW and MPR). We attended Duke University School of Medicine in the early 1960s and later served as house officers in the Department of Medicine. We knew Dr. Stead in the years before his retirement as chairman of that department in the time (we have been *told*, anyway) of his mellowing. We heard the stories of the other years. We walked the halls and worked the hours of those "iron men" of the '40s and '50s. Although we did not run into Dr. Stead at 2:00 A.M. on Osler or Long wards, nevertheless he was there.

Dr. Wyngaarden came in 1967 and it became his department. Yet Dr. Stead's tremendous influence remained. His colleagues have felt the need to keep the Stead tradition alive, to capture the essence of his wisdom. Perspicacity of Dr. Stead's thoughts is striking because of his ability to state complicated concepts in the simplest and often wittiest language. He is eminently quotable. Fred Schoonmaker and Earl Metz gathered 368 "Steadisms" into *Just Say For Me*, published in 1967. A further tribute was provided when Henry McIntosh, chief of the Duke cardiology division at that time, chaired a special committee which organized a symposium to honor Dr. Stead in 1968. The proceedings were published in the *Annals*, Volume 69, November 1968.

Dr. Stead appreciated the problems the new chairman would face. This was especially so since Dr. Stead was retiring from the chairmanship at the vigorous age of 59. His 20 years (1947–67) as a guiding force behind medical education at Duke had left its mark. An interruption was needed. So Dr. Stead accepted a Commonwealth Foundation fellowship and spent 12 months in New York City. He then returned to an office in a far corner of Duke Hospital. We were glad to have him back.

We were now better able to learn from him than before and have been changed by this experience. He has devoted himself to teaching and has performed an invaluable service as a sounding board for the young staff. We could not resist the urge to portray him in the total context in which we have known him.

There was yet another context, unique, developed during the 26 years in which Bess Cebe had worked for Dr. Stead. Together, they had administered a program which otherwise would have required a large support staff. With the addition of Bess, our editing group was complete.

We asked Dr. Stead's permission to use his writings, and his reaction went something like, "Well, that's not how I'd spend *my* time . . .," but he had no real objection. Later, as he saw the project shape up, he warmed to the idea. We hope that some day he will admit that he rather likes it.

Our illustrator is Alan Maver. GSW is a sports picture addict and had spent years searching for the Alan Maver who drew the sports cartoons which GSW had saved from his local newspaper as a boy. Alan worked from his home in Connecticut, using as source only the photographs from department files and from Dr. Stead's walls. We are fortunate to have found Alan Maver.

We have arranged our material into sections representing certain themes: the student years, the house staff years, the shaping of faculty, the business of being a doctor, et cetera. Within each section we have tried to preserve chronology, to illustrate the way Dr. Stead's philosophy about a certain issue evolved. To tell the truth, we haven't been able to discover a lot of evolution. Apparently Dr. Stead felt the same in 1947 about internship in community hospitals as in 1977. Through the years, he maintained that "what this patient needs is a doctor."

Mrs. Evelyn Stead is recognized as an essential factor in the E.A. Stead, Jr. equation. Annual gatherings of house staff and fellows at the Stead backyard 4th of July picnic, dinner parties for third-year students, picnics at the Lake for physical diagnosis students, and countless other amenities throughout the years were marked with her singular touch and graciousness. The children are Nancy, Lucy and Bill. At this writing, Nancy is on the Duke staff in hematology; Lucy is an excellent mother of two fine children; Bill is on the Duke staff in nephrology.

The reader is given a purview of Dr. Stead through his own words in Part I, "The Stead Philosophy." For those who would prefer first to find a review of his career, they may turn to Part II, "Biography." Part III places Stead in the context of the Duke Medical Center. The essays in this part, written by colleagues, are invaluable elements in the history of the medical school and hospital.

Like the Philosophy, the Biography is entirely in the words of Dr. Stead. Most material has been lifted from his various writings but in a few instances we asked him to write specifically to fill a gap in the story.

Throughout these chapters, we have attempted to place the quotations into sequences which relate to common concepts. Often, however, our task became complicated because a single comment provided insight into multiple concepts. Related ideas are separated by one bullet (•). When a complete change in direction occurs, we have used four asterisks (* * * *). Only those quotations which have been taken from published material have been footnoted. The remainder have been selected from his personal correspondence and addresses. Fred Schoonmaker, Bob Whalen, and Jay Skylar have kindly given us their own collections of Steadisms. The editors express their gratitude to many individuals who played important roles in the development of this book. O. William Jones, Noble David and Myrl Spivey have sent recollections of their days at Duke. John Furlow, Theodore Saros and Joe Sigler, of the Duke University staff, and Keith Sipe have provided sound advice on the preparation of the manuscript. Peggy Leggett, with the help of Dorothy Ellis, searched through the medical records to find the Osler ward rounding notes. Sidney Fortney, J.C. Gunnells, Ladd Hamrick, Douglas Kelling, Walter Kempner, O. William Jones, Robert McWhorter, Edward S. Orgain, Herbert O. Sieker, Myrl Spivey, Robert G. Sumner, and Robert Whalen have given us financial support for publication. Virginia Utley has assisted Bess Cebe in preparation of the manuscript. We especially appreciate the careful review and critique of the manuscript by Professor Irving B. Holley, professor of history, Duke University.

Preparation of *E.A. Stead, Jr.: What This Patient Needs Is a Doctor* has been an important and enjoyable experience for us. We express our final appreciation to Dr. Stead for being "the doctor."

Contents

Appendices

List of Plates

PART 1
THE STEAD PHILOSOPHY

The Terms of the Bond

TEACHING MEDICAL STUDENTS

No student will be flunked in his second year on the basis of any examination. If he has helped with the care of his patients, *the terms of the bond* are met. [editor's note: Under the new curriculum initiated in 1966, the student began clinical rotations in the second year.]

* * * *

The medical student's stimulus for learning is not to please his instructors but to give better service to his patients.

•

I have never tried to convert medical students into textbooks. If we did, we would clearly be forced to lower tuition since the best composite of medical knowledge can be purchased for about $150.[1]

•

I'd like to see all medical school examinations open book.[1]

The main thing to get out of medical school is a feeling of satisfaction with medicine. If so, the patterns developed will continue through life. It matters little the number of facts you accumulate in school.[1]

•

These students have met in classes and done exercises not related to any service function all of their lives. They need to be listened to, not talked to. They need to use words, handle ideas, discover the ways of building different houses from the same blocks, discover the noise in the communications system, and identify the differences between memory and thinking.[1]

* * * *

It is a neurotic goal to try and learn everything. One must pick and choose.[1]

•

Learning takes energy—so much so that I don't wish to learn anything without examining it in order not to have to unlearn it. I'm not ready to learn this now.[1]

•

One cannot be nervous about the student's ignorance. If he is learning one thing well, he is certainly not learning in many other areas. Our hope is that he will gain freedom and that he will learn to solve problems. The value of this program has to be evaluated in terms of fun and satisfaction. If the reward is considerable, the process will be repeated many times. If it is done only because the faculty requires it, the student might as well sleep throughout medical school. If he is going to sleep the rest of his life, no harm is done by taking a slight headstart in medical school.

•

Much of the learning on a clinical service goes on at night. The proper interaction within the student-intern-resident team is much more important than the senior staff-student interaction.

The student has never done anything for keeps. He needs to be given as much responsibility for patient care as he can assume, and this responsibility should be increased as rapidly as possible. Knowledge which is available for passing examinations is not available for daily use in clinical problems, and this conversion into useful knowledge will be achieved only by doing. His first responsibility lies to his patient. He will be physically present whenever any therapeutic or diagnostic procedures are being carried out, and he will take as active a part as his experience allows. This means that he will have the freedom to roam the entire medical center in pursuit of services to his patient.

Doctors have to give immediate care. Efficiency in history taking, physical examination, and relevant laboratory work is essential if the day's work is to be accomplished. He has to have enough patients to care for so that he learns this essential efficiency.

Students need to be relaxed and enjoy the real excitement of the hospital. They need to know that the faculty is aware that they cannot learn all clinical medicine in the second year. We want them to learn to think, and we will not be uneasy because they have not had time to examine every facet of medicine. When a student takes time to examine one clinical problem in depth, it goes without saying that he is not examining some other problem in depth. We will examine our student in the areas of his competence and not in his areas of ignorance. The areas of competence will be different in different students.

•

There's a difference between the observer's role and the participant's role. This becomes clear to me when I first step on a ward.[1]

•

The system of evaluation changes when the student enters the clinical area. Up until that time, he has made an A if he could answer the questions. In the clinical area, he is judged primarily by the effect of his actions on others. Is the day's work accomplished quicker and more pleasantly because he is there? Can he remember that the patients, the staff physician, the head nurse and the house staff have their own problems? Can he help solve some of these, or is he totally immersed in his own troubles? Can he do what needs to be done without being told? Does the patient regard him as a doctor? These qualities are even more important than answering examination questions directly.

•

[*Letter to chairman of another Department of Medicine*]: One of your students called us about summer school. I am not very enthusiastic about our own dull students and simply teach them as penance for my sins. Having lived a very upright life in the past year, I think I have done enough penance.

* * * *

In student ambulatory care teaching, only three things need to be accomplished: 1) increase the senior staff with primary outpatient responsibilities, 2) combine the time the student spends in the clinic into a single period, and 3) make it possible for a student to take his patient to a referral clinic and be seen more quickly.

In arranging the schedule to give the student more consecutive time in the outpatient clinic, certain facts should be kept in mind:

1) The senior year should not be all clinic work. When this is done, the student finds his senior year an anticlimax, with the third year the high spot in his medical school program.

2) The combined program of student and intern teaching which is effectively used by the department of medicine would break down if there were no senior students on the ward.

3) By leaving senior and junior students in the same area, the seniors obtain some of the satisfactions of teaching and the juniors have teachers they don't mind quizzing. Therefore, while I would like to increase the continuity of the student's clinical experience, I would not like to have senior students in the clinic the year around.

* * * *

We can teach basic science in the undergraduate colleges of the university, but we cannot teach medical science very effectively outside the medical school. Does the interplay between the basic scientist and the medical scientist in the research arena justify keeping the basic scientist in the medical school? I believe that it does.

I would open up the basic science courses in the medical school to science majors in the university instead of moving the basic scientists in the medical school back into the university. The courses taken in the medical school while in college would not have to be repeated in medical school. This would allow shortening of the traditional 8 years of medical school-college time.

A person going into a profession works at a different pace and with more purpose when he enters the domain where his life's work lies. As long as he is in the undergraduate college, most students adopt the familiar pattern of learning for the examination and then discarding the information as no longer useful. There is relatively little stimulus for the synthesis of broad areas of knowledge. This type of synthesis is the distinguishing mark of the medical student, in contrast to that of the more specialized graduate student.

*   *   *   *

There are many ways to teach and many ways to learn. I've always felt that it is important for a student to be on a ward early in his education so that he can see what doctors do and get a chance to manipulate his own ideas. Perhaps it would then be possible to later revisit the basic science area at a time when it would be more relevant.[1]

•

I've always felt that it is important in a curriculum to have available for a medical student a flexible period where he may spend time working with someone on the senior staff in depth, in order to learn quickly if he has any aptitude or interest in laboratory medicine.

•

One thing you need to know before you can get a good answer is what is the question.

•

I do not believe that any agreement should be made for required lectures in the second year of medical school without formal approval by the medical school advisory committee. Every medical school has its eyes on Duke. Can it make the core freshman year work? Can it resist the pressures of specialty areas such as radiology, community health sciences, dermatology, orthopedics, ophthalmology, et cetera, to convert back the second year to a sterile series of specialty areas?

The yielding to requests for required fixed points in the day for lectures in the second year will spell the death knell for the whole new venture. Let us not attempt to solve, in the same old way, the problems of clinical specialization which have broken the back of every attempted curriculum change to date. [1967]

•

Change is always more troublesome than sitting still. Change is most easily accomplished at the medical school-college interface or in the first two years of medical school. Innovation at this level will never have much effect on the educational program, because the majority of a doctor's education comes after that period of time. Any significant change will have to affect the clinical years of medical school, internship, residency and postgraduate education.

•

[*A colleague has requested Dr. Stead's approach to the student beginning clinical training*]: I usually make the following points:

Don't try to schedule time too tightly. Each patient has within him a story as exciting as one of Shakespeare's plays. Take the time to see the person who has the disease.

Learn to explore each new problem in depth. Consolidate your learning by teaching someone what you have learned. It makes no difference whether it is a nurse, a medical student, or your wife.

Keep a store of well-worked and used knowledge. Differentiate between the things that you know but can't be used by you in the middle of the night and the things that you both know and use. Continually increase the material usable by finding ways to put known but non-used material to work. Don't add supposed new facts to your store of worked-over knowledge until you have established that the new information is true and worth storing. Don't crud your crystal of usable knowledge.

Remember that your encounter with the patient can have three results. He may be better, he may be unchanged, he may be worse. Make a habit of collecting information over time so that you won't fool yourself or your patient.

Make as your educational goal the ability to care for patients in a way which makes each day worthwhile and enjoyable. Arrange the day so that there is little difference between work and play.

Don't try to cover your anxieties by compulsive behavior. You start your medical experience by being exceedingly thorough and careful. As time goes on, you discover in the care of each patient that some things are more important than others. The secret of success is to make the right selection each time.

* * * *

A doctor should regulate his conduct as he would expect a diabetic to regulate his insulin.[1]

•

[*Upon noting that a patient had erotic tendencies toward a student*]: Does she have other errors in judgment?

•

If you don't think you are going to make errors in clinical medicine you're not very bright, because the complexities are so great.[1]

•

I wouldn't criticize the bright guy who missed the diagnosis: we can all find times when we were that bright guy.

•

Analyze what it is by what it isn't.

•

It is particularly useful to the student to be encouraged to search the literature for references on the disease which he is treating. This helps one to realize that the material in books is often out of date.

•

Many facts are best left in books.

* * * *

The history can never be a mere mechanical recording of data. Each statement must be scrutinized for its possible bearing on the present status of the patient and, more particularly, for any light it may shed on the symptoms of which he now complains. The mind of a physician must be constantly alert to the possibility that any event related by the patient, any symptoms, however trivial or remote, may yet hold the key to the solution of the medical problem.[1]

•

From the history, one can usually estimate most accurately the speed of evolution of the disease. It is the taking of the history and in the analysis and interpretation of the data contained therein that the skill, knowledge and experience of the physician are most frequently and rigorously tested.[1]

•

I have a Dalmatian and everyone who comes over to my house and sees that dog says, "I know that dog from somewhere but can't place it." It's the same with students who have incomplete data.

•

Usually, diagnostic signs have been revealed because the observer has been prepared by other features of the history or examination to search for them.

•

It is impossible to educate or evaluate the confused; therefore I do a mental status early in the exam to see if I can rely on any of the data which follow.[1]

•

Regardless of the confusion of the data obtained from the history, regardless of the inconsistencies of statement voiced by the patient, the physical sign has an indisputable value as solid evidence.[1]

•

It's your murmur, you found it; so you tend to give it more significance.

•

Medicine isn't practiced without emotion. When I hear a murmur and you don't, I think it is a grade iii murmur. When you hear a murmur and I don't, I think it is a grade i murmur.

•

[*Re a lymph node*]: I like it because I found it.

* * * *

The student must learn both the liabilities and virtues of attempting to use logic in clinical medicine.

•

Most medical practice is not too tightly tied to science. The doctor must make decisions on the best available data and not be paralyzed by his ignorance. Many people cannot tolerate this uncertainty. The student needs to discover whether he thrives or atrophies in the clinical setting.

•

The art of medicine is not confined to organic disease; it deals with the mind of the patient and with his behavior as a thinking, feeling human being. The essential skills depend not simply on instruction but on emotional maturity manifest by sensitive self-cultivation of the ability to see deeply and accurately the problems of another human being. The challenge is further magnified by the fact that the examining physician is himself a human instrument, subject to error due to the events in his own biography.[1]

•

A doctor doesn't really need much knowledge, as he can look up most things. But he must have much emotional stability and ability to perform in an air of uncertainty.[1]

•

Doctors forget what they know over time, even though they become wiser. On Boards, the senior student is apt to do best.

•

Medicine is a service profession. The doctor agrees that patients can make demands on him—both reasonable and unreasonable—and that he will meet these needs. The student must determine whether he is comfortable with sick people, whether he can meet their multiple needs and still enjoy the day.

•

If you're going to enjoy the health professions, you have to develop a true tolerance for your fellow man.

•

A doctor is at the beck and call. If he worries about himself, he is not going to be a good physician. Staying up all night is only one of the hazards.[1]

There is clearly a difference between the physician who has doubts about his interest in clinical medicine and the physician who has doubts about his ability. I have always had much more patience with the latter.[1]

•

I am impressed each year by the great effort that medical students are willing to make. They have entered a profession for life, they see many doctors on the faculty obviously enjoying the fruits of their labor. First-year medical students at work are very different from college students at work. These differences provide the drive that causes two-year medical schools to evolve into four-year medical schools.

•

At the end of the second year the medical student will have satisfied all the terms of the bond. He is now free to differentiate in any way he likes.[2]

REFERENCES

1. Schoonmaker, F., Metz E. Just Say For Me. World Press Inc., Denver, 1968.
2. Stead, E. A. J. Med. Educ. **39**: 368, 1964.

To Care for the Person Who Has the Illness

HOUSE STAFF TRAINING

In the beginning you will care for the diseases that people have, but in time you will have mastered this phase of your work and you can care for the common diseases in your sleep. At that point, you will begin to become aware of the people who have the diseases and you will start *to care for the person who has the illness* as well as the illness itself.

•

Organic lesions have a way of compelling attention to themselves, and it is less exhausting to limit one's focus to this fear of organic disease. More time, energy and experience are necessary to view the patient as an active participant in an enormous moving pageant which includes the personal eccentricities of his forbears as well as the hopes for his children's future.[1]

•

I am sure that the patient should not be required to sign a permit while he is acutely ill. He has to know that his doctors are giving him the best of care.

•

I see no reason to remove from the patient the hope that he might do better; but you should let him know what the situation is by how you care for him.

•

The practical fact remains that the patient is embarrassed and the family is embarrassed by situations they are not familiar with. Help them.

•

I think it's very important that the family and the patient have the same information.

•

One interesting thing about all patients' behavior is that they want to behave like a good patient and good family should behave. We have to make clear to them how a good family should behave.

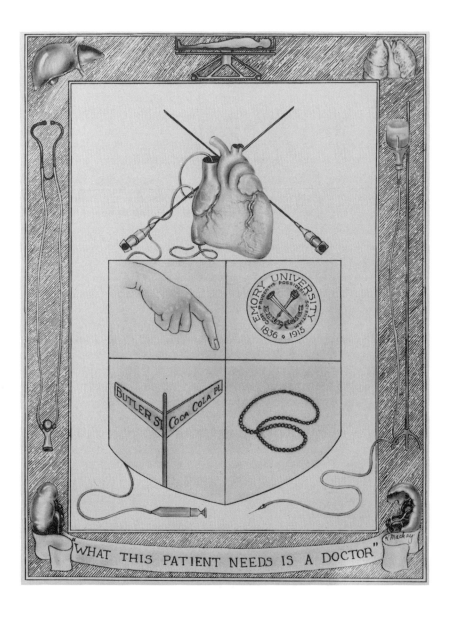

"WHAT THIS PATIENT NEEDS IS A DOCTOR"

•

A doctor ought to be able to tell when a dying patient has stopped suffering so that he can direct his attention to the suffering family.[1]

•

The medical profession is trained to save life. If a condemned criminal is hurt before the time for his execution, a team of doctors and nurses will work all night to keep him alive and restore his health.[2]

•

Getting out of this world gracefully is not an easy thing.

•

[*In re question of heart disease*]: She looks like a lady with unstable T-waves.

•

Everybody who has an ulcer is a person.

•

There's nothing wrong with giving the patient options and letting him elect what he wants.

•

Two things are important: one is to know that you don't know all the answers; the second is that when you divide patients into good and bad patients you'll find yourself rewarding the good patients and punishing the bad. So you should divide your patients into simple and complex ones.

•

The secret of handling hostility of the patient is to (1) not be hostile; and (2) let the patient talk about things.

•

I'm sure it is natural to feel hostility toward the "alcoholic." An amateur can feel any way he wants, but a doctor is a professional.[1]

•

Education does not make a man more tolerant. Some of the best educated people I have known have been the most intolerant.[1]

•

I never feel sorry for the doctor. The sick never inconvenience the well.[1]

•

Tact, sympathy and understanding are expected of the physician, for the patient is no mere collection of symptons, signs, disordered functions, damaged organs and disturbed emotions. He is human, fearful and hopeful, seeking relief, help and reassurance. To the physician, as to the anthropologist, nothing human is strange or repulsive. He cares for people because he cares for them.[1]

•

You let her know that she's a person and that you know how she feels and she'll respond better.

•

You must make any individual who is dying comfortable; what is comfortable depends on his culture and background.

•

The health professional has much more anxiety about dying than does the patient who is dying.

•

Sure, we can dramatically save your life, but then you'll go on and undramatically die of something else.

•

Pain is not the most distressing sympton to the dying. Nausea, vomiting, shortness of breath and dyspnea are, because physicians can't handle these as well.[1]

•

Pain can be relieved by narcotics; suffering is not touched by any drug I ever saw.

•

All disease sits in the substrate of a person: the soil in which things grow.

•

The restoration of the patient's comfort and confidence should begin with his initial contact with the physician and his assistants. Gentle, thorough and interested interrogation and examination prepare the way for more painful procedures that may be essential.[1]

* * * *

People are different. The less testing the more similarity, the more testing the less similarity.[1]

•

You need to look at the urine as hard when the patient is doing all right as you do when he isn't. Otherwise you won't know what to do with the information you get when he isn't.[1]

•

[*After a particularly prolonged effort to obtain specific information about laboratory results from a house officer, Dr. Stead's advice was*]: You should become more familiar with the Arabic culture. They have developed an interesting system; it is called numbers. You may find it useful to use this system as you go through life.

•

Most people tend to examine data for similarities. As a point of reference, I have enjoyed looking at the differences. In doing a physical examination, certain features of an illness may be obvious, but I have always had more fun looking for findings that make a given patient different from the other patients with that disease.[1]

•

In the practice of medicine the physician employs a discipline which seeks to use scientific methods and principles in the solution of its problems, but it is one which in the end remains an art. It is an art in the sense that rarely, if ever, can the individual patient be considered the equivalent of an experiment so completely controlled that it is possible to exclude judgment and experience from the interpetation of the patient's reaction.[1]

•

As I see it, doctors do three things: 1) subgroup the patient, 2) help the patient accept the subgroup, and 3) avoid trouble.

* * * *

The diagnostic procedure is a fascinating exercise. It involves the most acute use of our senses and the accurate recording of our observations. It requires the logical synthesis in the central nervous system of the responsible doctor, of information from the patient and his family, from other doctors who have cared for the patient in the past, from colleagues in various specialties who are helping with the immediate problem, and from the laboratory. Prognosis and correct therapy depend upon the correct use of the diagnostic process.

A diagnosis written in a record has an entirely different meaning. It consists of a single word or a few phrases. The person reading the diagnosis is supposed to be able to create in his mind's eye the entire clinical picture. The written diagnosis is the shorthand summary of the complete diagnostic procedure.

The diagnosis, as entered in the record, leaves out much of the information normally available during the diagnostic process. The assumption is made that all of the data have been collected accurately and interpreted correctly. The noise, which appears in all communication systems and which is inevitable when data are collected from multiple sources and persons of different competency, is disregarded.

The doctor in training will state that the patient was treated for an acute myocardial infarction three months ago. The doctor with experience will always ask: the diagnosis was supported by what data? He is interested in the setting of the illness, the experiences of the patient, the behavior of the doctor and the objective evidence to support the conclusion that some heart muscle died. The young doctor wants to conserve time by accepting the diagnosis of myocardial infarction. The older doctor wants to accumulate all available information and maintain as many options as possible. The young doctor can transmit his information in three words: acute myocardial infarction; but his chance of error-making is far greater.

. . . This problem of evaluating information and using it intelligently is common in any communication system. An object is spotted in the sky. It is identified as a hostile airplane (in our hypothetical patient, myocardial infarction). There is no difficulty in the transfer of information and the object is promptly shot down. If identification is deferred and all choices remain open, a tremendous amount of information must be continually transmitted and wide bands for communication must be available. The chance of a friendly airplane (or a significant medical finding) being destroyed because of error in identification is greatly decreased. When the choice is narrowed, the information is easy to transmit but the opportunity for error-making is increased. When all the information is transferred, the equipment required is complex, the dollar cost is high, but the error is reduced.

The transfer of information by the use of diagnostic terms is convenient shorthand and effective when the medicine is simple. When the medicine is hard, a review of the diagnostic procedures must replace the acceptance of the diagnosis.

The practice of medicine remains both fascinating and difficult.[3]

•

I always question in history-taking whether the inevitable should be left in or left out.

•

A lot of people get sick and, after a while, they just get well.

* * * *

If you do only a history, physical and laboratory evaluation, you rarely get information except that something exists. You need information about how much energy is stored in the system. And you need information of how much energy is spent by the system.

•

You have to recognize when the patient's central nervous system is no longer able to communicate with his fellow man; for all practical purpose he is then dead; only the heart and lungs continue to function.

•

Many nervous systems are capable of doing things that you think your nervous system wouldn't think possible.

You can only tell about what is going on in a patient's brain if you get playback from it. We can't make any assumptions. We can't believe we are communicating with a patient just by talking to him or at him. You must not be surprised when there are questions that you ask for which I have no dependable answer. That doesn't mean it's not a good question.

* * * *

In a way, interns are like patients with rheumatoid arthritis. Both have their limitations, and one has to learn to live with them.[1]

•

We don't really expect loyalty from our interns. In many cases, we didn't pick them and they didn't pick us. However, from our residents, who chose to stay with us, we do expect a high measure of loyalty.

•

The training of physicians is the purpose of the department of medicine at Duke University. Experience has taught us that the selection of your internship is the most important decision of your professional life. This experience will mold you more than any other. I am glad you are investing time in assessing the possibilities. As you examine our program, you must pay primary attention to our product. The details of how we produce the product will largely have to be taken on faith and, in all honesty, our judgment here will be better than yours. Do you have the capacity and desire to grow into the kind of person we produce? Duke is not for everybody, and medicine is a demanding mistress. Experience has shown that Duke does give a very rewarding experience to intelligent graduates who wish to achieve excellence in medicine.

To accomplish this our staff 1) takes care of patients: sick and well, poor and rich, educated and uneducated; 2) engages in research at many levels; and 3) teaches a wide variety of students. Our prime product is not the care of patients or the production of new knowledge by research. Men are our prime product—men to care for sick and well patients; men to do medical research; men to carry out the varied functions needed by the health field. Responsibility for patient care, participation in the teaching program, and close contact with a staff engaged in patient care, research and writing are the essential ingredients for a program charged with producing trained manpower.

The medical internship and residency program at Duke is designed to give to the intern a knowledge of the factual material in the field of medicine and a sound philosophical basis for a lifetime of learning in practice. What is done is important, but why it is done is even more important. Duke is not just a collection of excellent doctors. It is a group of doctors who have carefully thought out a program of training which will allow maximum growth of people. The staff does believe that doctors exist to care for people. It does believe that patients can legitimately make demands on doctors and that, because the ill are not rational, these demands do not have to be rational. The staff does believe that the practice of medicine has many emotional and intellectual rewards. It believes that the intellectual rewards of practice can be combined with economic rewards if the physician has learned to care for private patients in a teaching atmosphere. Research and private care can be carried on simultaneously if opportunities have been available for this kind of learning during the training period. The staff believes that there are many pitfalls in learning in the multivariable, ill-characterized systems typified by the patient.

The Duke faculty puts many hours of work into both graduate and undergraduate training. One-half of our interns are usually Duke graduates. This means that when you come to Duke you join a team which has already begun to understand the why's of the program in the department.

Interns, residents and undergraduate students work in our public wards and public clinics, in our private wards and private clinics, in our Veteran's Hospital and on an elective basis in our research laboratories. We have a single faculty staffing these facilities. The third- and fourth-year student, the intern and the first-year resident form a close working unit for purposes of learning how to care for patients and for learning how to learn in a system as complex as the patient. Everyone in this unit is both a teacher and a learner. Learning is an active process and each of us learns more when we teach than when we are taught.

Some of our doctors from other schools are surprised at the emphasis we place on the fact that they must teach. They say that since more of our interns will practice than will remain in the university, this emphasis may be misplaced. We take the opposite point of view. The practitioner does more teaching than the academician. The physician in practice teaches his office personnel, his paramedical assistants and, above all, his patients. The noise in the information transfer systems, the twist given to one word which inverts the whole concept, the differences in the intake systems of two different persons, these are the same whether the intern is trying to teach the student, or the doctor is trying to teach a diabetic patient to live with his disease.

The intern year is a year of doing. The intern must handle a volume of work great enough to make him become efficient in giving medical care. The volume of work must be great enough to make him selective. He cannot solve his problem by devoting an equal amount of time to each area of the examination. He must explore and rapidly discard the irrelevant areas, but spend as much time as need be on the relevant areas. He will make errors. The staff will pick up these errors and prevent harm to the patient. The next time around, the intern will make the right decision.

The intern, as the do-er, must be fed intellectually by the student below and by his first-year resident above. By the end of the year he will be comfortable with any patient with any illness. All the rest of his life he will give patient care quickly and efficiently. Each day, his intern training will give him time for other ventures. The intern year requires a large investment of time and effort, but it guarantees continued dividends.

The third and fourth years of the undergraduate school, the internship and first-year residency are devoted to teaching the doctor how to care for and to understand people—sick and well. At the end of this time he appreciates the complexity of the problems in clinical medicine; he understands how to set up learning situations as he cares for patients; and he understands the integrated behavior of the organism in which disease processes may occur. Under the guidance of the clinical staff, he has re-read his physiology, pathology, biochemistry, pharmacology, anatomy and microbiology. He has made the connections in his brain between clinical and preclinical learning. He is now ready to learn more about the special procedures which are useful in medicine. If he wishes to specialize, he may carry this out in many ways. He may spend one or more years working with specialists in the area of their special competence. He may spend a year rotating through several specialties. He may go to the laboratory to master some of the areas of science which underlie the practice of medicine. He may work out a year of combined clinical and laboratory experiences. There are, then, many ways to use the Medical Center after the internship and first-year residency. We work out specialized programs to fit the diverse needs of our men. We try to structure programs to use effectively the years committed to required government service. Productive use of this time is more important than any particular sequence of training. We always take back at any time our residents who have their programs interrupted by call to service.[4]

•

It is very hard to go home and think great thoughts when you are bone tired from being in the clinic or operating room all day long.

* * * *

In a rotating service the intern is responsible to the hospital and to the intern committee. He has avoided making a commitment to any one area, but he has usually identified one or two areas in which he has little interest. When he is assigned to these services, he does not pull his weight.

. . . There are many definitions of a teaching hospital. I have always said that a teaching hospital is one in which the intern and resident can teach, rather than one in which they are taught. Medical students are the greatest single asset of a teaching hospital. Properly woven into the program, they give the intern and resident the opportunity for an active participation in the learning, which can come only from establishing correlation between biologic processes and disease, from the manipulation of ideas and from the painting of word pictures. I know of many ways to teach medical students without the use of interns and residents as teachers. I know of no method of intern and resident training that is as effective as one that involves them directly in the teaching program.

. . . As advanced students of clinical medicine, interns and residents of necessity perform some service. What should they be paid? The idea of paying them primarily for service has never been seriously proposed for one simple reason: the intern and resident can create more funds by practice than the hospital can collect for their services. Even if 100% of the income created by the residents were returned to the residents they would still be underpaid.

As advanced students of clinical medicine, they require a faculty and appropriate library and laboratory facilities. They cannot possibly create enough income to pay for the cost of their education.[5]

•

House officers once made no money and incurred no debts, therefore they were stable. Today they are making more money and incurring more debts and are more unstable.[1]

•

An employer receiving services from his employees should pay a wage comparable to services received. An educational institution teaching graduate students has to pay a faculty. It will supply the best scholarship for the students that it can, but it will not seek to pay wages. Any intern or resident working for wages should be given some other title, to indicate that he is employed for service.

•

Many persons believe that the internship and residency are designed as a period of supervised practice and that, during this period of supervised work, the resident should be exposed to every clinical problem he will ever have to solve. Those with this philosophy structure their programs so that the residency experience is as much like practice as possible. I believe Dr. _____ would belong to this very honorable school of thought.

I have always looked on the residency years as preparation for the continuing education which should take place during practice, and I have structured our program to be as unlike practice as possible.

. . . To be an effective physician one must be able to give of himself without resentment. Patients must be free to make demands on him when they are socially least attractive.[6]

•

I can always tell how a junior resident is progressing by how he handles the situation when all the laboratory tests are negative. A good intern knows what to do when the laboratory results are positive.

•

A city hospital trains people for disease, not for learning about people.[1]

•

Two years in a hospital, night and day, are necessary to see how illness looks—to see what the people behind the patient look like in all circumstances.[1]

•

A hospital is a service institution. It is difficult for me to understand why house officers are afraid to see patients admitted. I've never been afraid of any patient.[1]

•

If you can't get your work done in 24 hours, you'd better work nights.[1]

* * * *

Our senior assistant residents rotate through the various clinical specialties, not so much to learn specific techniques but to make the discovery that none of the techniques used by the specialists are particularly difficult and that they can be learned by them whenever they see enough patients of a particular type to make it desirable to invest the time for learning them.

•

A senior resident too often wants to be smart and not helpful.

•

The chief resident is the chief doctor among so many experts. Like Churchill, he's not the brightest in any field but knows where and how to seek help when necessary.

•

I've never seen an efficient house officer; with very few exceptions, it is a time to be inefficient.

•

In our medical school I always assume that our graduates will take care of sick and well people. No amount of research aptitude or interest expressed by the man in training persuades us that he will not eventually doctor. The rewards, emotional and intellectual, of doctoring are too high.[6]

•

[*Re need for surgery*]: Most young men would take it out. I myself would get an old doctor. The final decision will be emotional and not scientific.

•

Sometimes an old, very ill patient needs to have a doctor who is not a good doctor.

•

[*Words Make Pictures*]: If I want to communicate with you, I have to have some way to form pictures in my mind and send them to you. In turn I must have the means to reconstruct pictures in my mind from material you send me. The only way to evaluate the communication which has actually occurred is for you to sketch out the material you have received and for me to sketch out the material I have sent. There are many possibilities for error making in the communication system and one function of the teacher is to be certain that the sources of error are always near the level of consciousness. This is particularly important for the physician in practice because teaching patients about health and illness is so important a part of his daily life. The academician can afford to make errors because his students are more likely to correct him.

We all know that we cannot avoid the noise in the communication system between two persons by having them both examine the same picture. For years I have asked doctors to draw a detailed picture of an optic fundus we have both examined. Knowing how unlikely one is to make an accurate reproduction, I have usually asked them to label the sketch either "1" or "2". "One" means that they have drawn the fundus as it isn't. "Two" indicates that they have drawn it as it is. Regardless of which way they initially label the sketch, they usually end up by suggesting it be labelled "1". A person unskilled in communication would be trapped into believing that both central nervous systems had created the same image because both eyes had looked at the same thing.

The most common way to communicate is by words. The sender conveys the picture in his brain into a series of symbols which he says or writes. These symbols (words) are received by the ears or eyes of another person. He decodes them by creating a picture in his central nervous system. If the sender makes an error in transcription and uses a word that does not convey accurately that portion of the picture the word is supposed to symbolize, noise enters the communication system and the receiver will not be able to construct a clear picture. If the sender uses a word for which he has no picture (a word that he cannot accurately define), he is not participating in communication. He is carrying out non-communication. It is surprising how many words used by college graduates are non-communicating symbols. I have learned this by asking generations of students to define words. They make my ears red from time to time by catching me indulging in non-communication. Nevertheless, because I am interested in communication, I win most of the nickels.

If I transcribe my picture correctly into symbols, I may still be in trouble. The person receiving the symbols may not receive all of them. There may be trouble in the receiving set of the type exemplified by color blindness. The person may never receive all the information I have offered him. If he does receive all the symbols, he may not have the information to assemble them to form the same picture that I have sent. One or more of my words may create no portion of my picture. This difference may be in content or it may be in the size of the objects or the brilliance of the color. The only way to tell what I tried to send and what he received is for each of us to sketch out the picture and then compare it detail by detail. It will surprise you how often the receiver draws the non-picture instead of the picture.

Some persons are intuitively more conscious of the relationship between words and imagery. These persons are vocal, expressive and communicative. They are apt to have an odd view of the world because they assume that other people are the same way. As a doctor, I've been struck many times by the lack of imagery in many persons' lives. They form few pictures and talk little.

It is very important for the doctor to know what the patient has learned. He can discover this only by having the patient create pictures for the doctor to examine. It is useful to have the patient describe his illness and the prescribed treatment. He will have to define the pictures created by words which may be still strange to him. It will be surprising to note how often he creates the non-treatment picture rather than the treatment picture.[7]

•

When I get up in the morning I brush my teeth, eat and walk to the hospital. I don't like to do these things but I have to do them—the same for the history meeting.

REFERENCES

1. Schoonmaker F, Metz E. Just Say For Me. World Press Inc., Denver, 1968.
2. Stead EA. Medical Times 95: 1173, 1967.
3. Stead EA. Medical Times 95: 588, 1967.
4. Stead EA. Medical Times 94: 1001, 1966.
5. Stead EA. New England J. Med. 269: 240, 1963.
6. Stead EA. Pharos of AOA 29: 70, 1966.
7. Stead EA. Medical Times 96: 1249, 1968.

DUKE · UNIVERSITY
SCHOOL · OF · MEDICINE

THIS · IS · TO · CERTIFY · THAT

Eugene A. Stead Jr., M.D.

HAS · COMPLETED · CREDITABLY
IN

DUKE HOSPITAL

Chief of Medical Services
10 Years

DURHAM, N.C.
MAY 6, 1957

SAMUEL P. MARTIN	'47
BERNARD C. HOLLAND	'48
JAMES F. SCHIEVE	'49
GRACE P. KERBY	'50
JAMES W. HOLLINGSWORTH	'51
GERALD RODNAN	'52
HARRY McPHERSON	'53
MORTON BOGDONOFF	'54
SUYDAM OSTERHOUT	'55
DONALD MERRITT	'56

DUKE · UNIVERSITY
SCHOOL · OF · MEDICINE

THIS · IS · TO · CERTIFY · THAT

Eugene A. Stead Jr., M.D.

HAS · COMPLETED · CREDITABLY
IN

DUKE HOSPITAL

Chief of Medical Services
Next 10 Years

DURHAM, N.C.
JUNE 1967

JOHN V. VERNER	'57
ARNOLD M. WEISSLER	'58
ROBERT E. WHALEN	'59
HOWARD K. THOMPSON	'60
CHARLES E. MENGEL	'61
T. DAVID ELDER	'62
ANDREW G. WALLACE	'63
MICHAEL E. McLEOD	'64
EARL N. METZ	'65
HARRY M. CARPENTER	'66

The Chief Residents, Duke

3

"Thinking Ward Rounds" Are Useful

SAMPLES OF NOTES WRITTEN DURING
OSLER WARD ROUNDS 1947–77

How do you learn to think? One way is to practice. But what do you practice and in what setting? One way is to have ward rounds which are pointed specifically at thinking.

The learning process can be divided into the accumulation of bits of information (memory) and the movement of these bits into patterns which are new to the individual (thinking). A little reflection will make it clear that the compulsive learner is incapable of thinking. There is always another bit to be memorized and, if they are all learned, there is little time to rearrange the bits in original patterns. It is also clear that without any bits there is no thinking. The hardest theoretical question in educational circles is the determination of the optimum number of bits for the most effective manipulation.

Problem solving may or may not involve thinking. If one reads another person's solution to a problem, the answer is acquired through memory and no manipulation of data is achieved. If one solves a problem by the application of a known routine or formula, no thinking is required. One may obtain a solution to the problem of 98 multiplied by 7 without doing any thinking. On the other hand, solution of a problem by the rearrangement of bits of information into patterns that are new to the individual is, by definition, thinking. An attempt to solve a problem by thinking frequently serves as a stimulus to accumulating new bits of information. The addition of new bits may suddenly allow combinations of old and new memorized material to be arranged in patterns novel to the individual.

Now for thinking ward rounds. A patient is seen who has a record of nocturia. Careful questioning establishes that the patient does not have frequency from irritation of the bladder or from neurological disease and does not have to wake to void because of a large amount of fluid imbibed shortly before bedtime or during the night. The patient, in fact, drinks normally during the day but, as recorded in his history, he excretes at night an abnormally increased volume of urine. Why is this information useful to the doctor? Identify a common denominator relating to the phenomenon of nocturia, the metabolic disturbance in thyrotoxicosis, and Cheyne-Stokes respiration associated with a greatly enlarged heart. Relate the generalization derived to the practice of medicine.

The next few minutes are spent in being certain that the problem is properly recorded. The information to be collected about nocturia, about thyrotoxicosis and about certain forms of Cheyne-Stokes breathing can be likened to the learning of arithmetic and involves mainly memory. The generalization which relates these three commonly observed clinical problems is not found in textbooks and one must convert the specific knowledge gleaned from a more perceptive look at the three syndromes into some more useful generalization. In mathematics, this would be changing from the arithmetic that $2 + 2 = 4$ to the algebraic generalization that $a + b = c$.

The matter is then re-opened after several days. Several solutions may be derived but none can be achieved without thinking.

This formulation appeals to me most. The usual sequence of drinking is well known to any beer hall keeper. He supplies large amounts of liquid and ample toilet facilities. His experience shows: beer in=beer out, no nocturia. Our patient had uncoupled a normally well-coupled system and the uncoupling was revealed by the presence of increased water output at night without any increased fluid intake during the night. The clinically useful information is that a normally closely coupled sequence has become uncoupled.

In thyrotoxicosis, food is burned with the production of ATP. In the normal subject the burning of substrates for energy is coupled to the process of phosphorylation. As ATP accumulates, the metabolic fires are banked. In thyrotoxicosis, a tightly coupled system has become uncoupled. Substrate utilization is not inhibited by normal concentrations of ATP and the amount of substrate burned is no longer related to the amount of ATP present.

In Cheyne-Stokes respiration with a big heart, the O_2 and CO_2 concentrations of the blood entering the left heart may be greatly different from the concentrations of these gases in blood leaving by the aorta. During hyperpnea, the heart empties itself of dark blood accumulated during the previous period of apnea and at the same time fills itself with well-oxygenated blood with a low CO_2 content. The nervous system continues to respond to the unoxygenated blood with a high CO_2 content until all the black blood is gone and the heart is filled with red blood. Apnea occurs as the oxygenated blood is delivered to the nervous system and a chemical stimulus for breathing will be absent until all the red blood is emptied from the heart. During the period of apnea, the heart is being filled from the unventilated lungs. Again a tightly coupled system relating the concentrations of these gases in arterial blood has become uncoupled.

The algebraic generalization is that symptoms of illness obvious to both the patient and the doctor will develop when reactions which are normally coupled become uncoupled.

The goal of such an exercise is to improve the ability to think. Exercises related to patient care must be devised which involve thinking. The student deserves concrete illustrations of the thinking process. *Thinking ward rounds are useful.*[1]

SAMPLES OF NOTES WRITTEN BY DR. STEAD DURING
HIS OSLER WARD ROUNDS 1947–1977

I think the problems of living are going to be the only problems we modify.

•

The patient feels well, better today, and well may have begun to improve. We cannot settle the cause between homologous serum jaundice and infectious hepatitis. The complications of confinement to bed are greater than the complications of getting out of bed.

•

The only solution I know to this is patience.

•

I assume the immediate symptoms are the manifestation of a diabetic neuropathy. The first therapeutic move would be an enema.

•

The iron deficiency is most obvious thing to treat. I think a small intestinal biopsy would be of interest. I suspect he will never be free of GI symptoms. The key to the problem may be to convince him that he is not ill.

•

His hospitalization should be made as short as possible because of his night job and diabetes. I am not sure he has profited by his insulin change. He says his socks no longer become moist.

•

It would be nice if this man could be induced to cease his alcohol ingestion.

•

I detect no evidence of localized vascular disease. The cogwheel rigidity of Parkinsonism and the effects of the demerol suggest an inelastic central nervous system.

•

I have nothing to add. Patient says she is feeling better and her chart seems to agree with this.

•

I think he has had an idiopathic epilepsy and, as he is unable to function to support his family, I would be cautious about adding any more loads than necessary.

•

I have no specific notions about therapy. I suspect he will benefit more by the nonspecific functions of the hospital.

•

I find nothing in the history or physical exam to indicate the nature of his trouble. He remarried a year ago and has never held a job more than 2½ years and has usually stopped because of being bored. In addition to his stomach complaint, he complains of weakness and nervousness. We have a clear indication for a thorough examination of the kidneys, gallbladder and entire GI tract including pancreas, but I do not know if we will find anything abnormal.

•

I see no reason not to try out the pacemaker but I am not wise enough to know how this will alter his activity.

•

The story is more that of gastritis than of ulcer. It is clear that, if he continues to live as he does, he will have stomach trouble.

•

I would be cautious as to the use of pressor agents and try her off them now. If that doesn't work, put her back on them.

•

Dr. Cook points out an aberrant shadow on x-ray which he interprets as a vein. This interpretation appeals to me.

•

The relation of the pain to motion and cough does not sound like coronary artery disease. I am not certain why she comes to the hospital. It would appear that many of her admissions have been on the basis of house staff anxiety.

•

He does have rheumatoid arthritis. He has given up. Let's see what we can do for him.

•

I have no notion what caused his head edema and I would not favor making him sick with drugs.

•

His incapacitation probably relates to his I.Q. and not sarcoid.

•

I think we are in a situation where acceptance of the illness is better than a cure.

•

[Re patient, admission # 3]: Our immediate problem is treating her acute asthmatic attack. Our real problem is teaching this girl how to deal with life.

•

[Same patient, admission #12]: The immediate problem is treating her acute asthmatic attack. The real problem is teaching her how to deal with life.

•

[Same patient, admission #13]: The immediate problem is well cared for. The solution to the chronic problem is not clear.

•

We have a difficult problem with the combination of asthma and infection, weight loss, depression and desire for industrial compensation.

•

I detect no evidence of localized pathology in the neck. The circulation is very hyperactive and, for this reason, I am not very likely to interpret a supraclavicular thrill as very meaningful. Indeed, the temperature combined with amenorrhea would lead me to examine the pelvis.

•

In view of the acuteness of the hypertension and the fact that he has a few areas of local narrowing in the eyes, I would probably push the workup to the point of arteriogram. I would make every effort to change his picture of patients and doctors.

•

Her pattern is that of a person with a sensitive nervous system in whom the symptoms have been more dramatic in the side. If we can obtain a physician to take care of her more completely, we'll see more progress.

•

I do not feel the thyroid; trachea is somewhat deviated to the right. I hope Drs. Broughton and Hunn will examine available data and come to the proper conclusions.

•

Clinical course to date has not been overwhelmingly successful. Our question is whether to do more of same or look for other ways to alter the illness. I have no strong reactions.

•

We have the interesting problem of sensation produced from the gut not protected by the stomach in an individual with a central nervous system. As is customary, the attempt to solve this by drugs has failed. I will be interested in Dr. McDaniel's solution to the problem.

•

The acute drug problem has been satisfactorily cared for and we are now faced with the problem of treating the patient.

•

I believe the hypertrophy and dilatation of the left ventricle is from 1) chronic anemia, 2) hard work of coughing, 3) raising 10 children.

•

I agree that Dr. Temple is smart enough to take care of this woman.

•

We have the familiar problem of organic illness, aging, limited education. My question is whether we can ever make this man productive.

•

The obesity dominates the picture. It is difficult to think of a therapeutic approach that doesn't involve lightening the weight on his feet and on his metabolic process.

•

The problem is one of adaptation to the present machine rather than changing the machine.

•

It would be most fun if he had a left atrial myxoma.

•

This patient is a good example of the interplay of those symptoms which are coronary in origin and those which are not coronary in origin.

•

The patient's circulation is overactive and raises the familiar question of why.

•

The inability to repress nervous activity is outstanding.

•

The most impressive thing this morning is his bladder, which is visible. I am curious as to whether he can empty it. I would try to study it with x-ray rather than catheter.

•

The symptomatology is diffuse and clearly reflects his opinion that he is not employable and therefore I would have no objection to certifying him for Social Security.

•

She should know as much as possible about gonorrhea as she will probably meet this problem again.

REFERENCES

1. Stead EA. Medical Times **95**: 706, 1967.

• 4 •

We Produced No Single Product

DEVELOPMENT OF MEDICAL MANPOWER

I tried to determine the best fit in life, in helping a large number of students and residents work out their career pattern. These doctors were all different; *we produced no single product*. We were a busy workshop where differentiation into many forms was possible. We honored the man who did excellent general practice as much as the specialist, research scientist, and doctor with administrative talents.

•

Students, interns and residents come to us for training. Each is different and each gains satisfaction in a different way. Our role is not to stamp out residents from a common mold. Our goal is to identify the best use of the man and to find the limits imposed by his structure.[1]

•

One of the ways of judging a man is deciding whether he is worth the trouble he creates. If he is very productive, we can tolerate a lot of trouble. If he is not overly productive, he had better be a nice fellow.

•

You can't judge a man at any one point in time. You have to look at his growth curve. As long as his curve is up, there is no way of predicting where his productivity will stop.

•

I don't have much trouble dealing with aggressive people. I find it easy to get out of their way. It is much harder dealing with lazy people, because I have never found out how to get them moving.

•

We examine the language requirements for reading the relevant literature. We find the language deficit more commonly related to symbolic language of mathematics, physics, chemistry, electronics and engineering than to French, German or Russian.

•

Education in medicine or anything else is just a way of becoming a free man. The more competent you become, the more opportunity you have to do as you please.[1]

•

I have always liked the story of the tortoise and the hare since there is no ceiling on man's growth and since learning curves are so different.[1]

•

One way for the student to learn the difficulties in drawing accurate conclusions about biological systems is to give him the opportunity to establish some fact on the basis of his own work. We call this research and find it a very effective method of teaching. The intellectual discipline involved better prepares him for the role of a lifetime learner.

•

An unwillingness to listen and test one's present feelings against those of others is somewhat like burning books.

* * * *

Consideration of the state of medical education reveals a remarkable sameness from school to school and from year to year. Most medical school faculties have had similar educational backgrounds because a relatively small group of schools sired most of those who have become the major decision-makers in our medical schools and because like begets like. Medical faculties are remarkably unsophisticated about the latent potentialities of working with different mixes of faculty, students and subjects, because all of their lives have been spent in recycling a single type of student through relatively fixed programs.

•

The physician has the opportunity to modify his brain and make it a more flexible instrument by using it to solve problems posed by those concerned with furthering knowledge in health fields. In the past, we have used the learning of bioscience as the primary means of modifying the student's nervous system. The uninitiated have thought that the content of these sciences was essential to the practice of medicine, but the more sophisticated have realized that the reward for such study was an overall increase in competence of the nervous system and was not directly related to the subject matter.

* * * *

One can quickly sense the interest of a specialty area giving education in depth if one discusses the internship and service time with the chief of the service. If the chief will accept any type of internship and any type of service experience as adequate preparation for his residency program, one should avoid him as one would the plague.

All physicians can have a role in these projections into the future. In our medical centers, the fulltime teachers are apt to take the lead—not because they are brighter or more capable but because they are paid in such a way that they have the leisure time for thinking.

In order to carry out our program effectively, we have to have a flow of patients through our department, and we have to give effective care to these patients. A medical school by definition teaches patient care. We try to make this care excellent and, from the beginning, to use the needs of the patient as the stimulus for learning. We need many kinds of patients: those with acute illness, those with chronic illness, and those with acute exacerbations of chronic problems, those with wealth and education as well as those with overwhelming poverty and illness. We prefer the service not to be too submerged with patients who can no longer work and who require a large amount of mechanical work from the service. We wish to be able to see the person with illness as well as the illness.

* * * *

Educational programs in community hospitals are rarely successful. They are commonly modeled after university medical centers. Because the functions and financing of the university medical center and the community hospital are widely different, it is not surprising that the transplanted program does not flourish in the new environment.

The medical center receives funds to support the time which the faculty spends in teaching and training. It also supports the time the faculty spends in the laboratory and library preparing for its teaching duties. The university medical center can, therefore, make the expensive investment in time required for converting untrained personnel into a highly skilled product.

The community hospital is a user of the skilled personnel produced by the university medical center. The professional staff of the community hospital gives service to the community. The demands for service are so great that the physician has little time for contemplation and postgraduate education. Any program of training or teaching put into the community hospital which requires an investment of professional time makes matters worse. The last bits of thinking time disappear with the assumption of additional teaching. A teaching service is added to an already heavy patient-service load.

It is not surprising that community hospital educational programs falter when they attempt to teach new classes of interns and residents each year. With a great effort, the staff spends time with the residents only to discover that they do this at the expense of their last leisure moments. They do not have the time to both prepare for their teaching activities and then to perform them.

The community hospital is a place where physicians give services to people. Money is not available to support a large portion of the staff to interact with students, interns and residents and to pay for the increase in cost of services, which is unavoidable where service is one of the devices for converting green manpower into trained manpower. The staff of the community hospital is responsible for care in the office, in the home, in the nursing home and extended care units, and in the hospital. The most precious commodity in the doctor's life is time. An internship and residency program in the community hospital saps up the last vestige of time. The doctor attempts to educate the intern and resident, but he soon discovers that he does not have the time to continue his own education. After a tremendous effort, the educational program usually gives little satisfaction to the doctor, to the patient, to the hospital, or to the intern and resident.

During my time as chairman of the departments of medicine at Emory and Duke, I never urged my students to take internships and residencies in community hospitals. The staff of the community hospital is concerned with medicine as it is practiced today. The internship and residency are golden years in which one can learn both the medicine of today and the language and theoretical underpinning of the medicine of tomorrow. No community hospital has the faculty to combine these two elements: the best practice of today and the best preparation for the practice of tomorrow. . . . My own observations indicate that the fathers practicing medicine in community hospitals that ask to be supplied with interns advise their own sons to take their graduate training in a medical center closely tied in with a university and with undergraduate training.

•

I have a great interest in developing new programs and patterns in community hospitals. I have no interest at all in attempting to shore up existing programs which I believe are certain to fail.

•

If I were going to work in this area, I would try two approaches. I would 1) increase the skilled help in the hospital with trained male physician assistants, 2) obtain the time for the educational program by building office facilities as a part of the hospital. The staff, by using the hospital laboratories for its outpatient work, could support the office building. The saving in time by devoting one's entire working day in one area would create time for thinking.

•

I have no question at all that time is the most valuable asset the internist has and that he pays a high price if his professional life is not effectively organized.

•

The key problem is how to return some free time for thinking to the professional staff of the community hospital.

* * * *

Learning is an active process and each of us learns more when we teach than when we are taught.

•

The mistake made by the young teacher is in thinking that the student is receiving, grasping and learning all that is presented. This is corrected by hearing the playback. Increased teaching equals decreased learning for the student.

•

I've always thought that the best teacher placed the least limitation on his students. He set the pattern for fun and satisfaction and inspired continued learning after he had disappeared. Finally, he must make himself dispensable so that the student can grow up and become independent of him.

•

Clinical departments need teachers to help in transferring to their students information present in books. They need, also, teachers who are going to present to the student a clear picture of what is not known about biological systems and who can inspire and lead the student to prepare himself to solve some of these puzzling and interesting problems.

As they teach their colleagues, they learn that each person has a personalized receiving system and an individualized processing system. They make the discovery that they can never predict the effect of any input into the nervous system of another man by any form of theoretical calculation. They have to listen to the playback from the system receiving the input to determine the degree of change produced. This information is of incalculable value in the practice of medicine.[3]

•

Teaching should be the price of admission to the club and not something to be paid for over the period in which you belong to the faculty. Teaching should be for love and not for pay. The teaching budget should pay for time over and beyond that contributed by the average faculty member, but each man so supported should know that over his lifetime he cannot expect major support from the teaching budget.

•

An occasional man will break the mold. When that happens, enjoy him but do not build your house on this unlikely-to-be-found rock.[3]

•

Effective teaching is an interaction and can be prevented by the student, teacher or both.

•

The teacher is most useful when the student is active. The more active the teacher, the less the learning opportunity for the student.

•

How can one identify the long-lived teachers and thus avoid the boredom present in many schools? Select those who are more interested in conveying attitudes than in transmitting facts. Select those who are more concerned with what is not known about a subject than in the transmission of current knowledge. Select those who listen well rather than those who parrot the same record each time the button is pushed. Select those who, as a matter of pride in their own ability, listen carefully to define areas for intellectual exploration when the resident says, "this patient is of little interest". Select those who do not take themselves too seriously and are willing to be replaced by able youngsters, realizing that eventually they must become less important to the institution. Select those who require excellence from their students at all times. Effort and good intentions are not enough. Select those who are happy teachers and who will die for only certain things. Most of the time they will walk around obstructions and not bloody their noses unnecessarily. Select those who share with students the fun and satisfaction created by the intellectual achievement of the student. The returns to the student for his efforts create enough pleasurable feelings for him to want to repeat the process. Select those who best understand the limitations of teaching. Select those who can tolerate ignorance.

The most effective teachers create a shadowy framework in which the student can climb. If the teacher fills in the skeleton in great detail, he will limit the learning by his own knowledge. If he makes the form recognizable but leaves the final shape and details to the student, the student may produce a much better intellectual synthesis than the teacher. A teacher may be likened to an artist. A pedestrian artist may produce an exact copy of a scene and most viewers will see approximately the same thing. The picture will not live because it will have little relevance to the changing patterns of life. A much less precise picture, suggesting a mother and child which leaves many details to the imagination, will come to life in as many interpretations as there are viewers. Some of these interpretations may be superior to the original concept of the artist. [1968]

* * * *

On any clinical service, one finds a number of bright young residents who are very effective teachers of the current state of the art. They are capable doctors, completely trustworthy and loved by both patients and students. They are interested in what is known. They have nothing which they want to contribute to extend existing knowledge, and they have no stimulus to use scientific journals to communicate with their colleagues.

When we allow these currently effective teachers to move into practice without marked effort to hold them in the university, we are severely criticized by our students at both the undergraduate and graduate level. We are accused of killing off teachers by the "publish or perish" attitude. We are told that we should reward good teaching by academic tenure, early promotion and good pay.

I have never believed that it is desirable to add a person to the permanent faculty because he is a good and effective teacher.

When we add a man to our faculty, we make a lifelong commitment. If we select him primarily for his teaching ability, we have decided to use him as a teacher for the duration of his life. We have selected him not for his other attributes but for this teaching ability. The problem inherent in this basis of selection is in the fact that few teachers remain maximally effective as teachers over their full professional lifetime.

Since students are undergoing continual change, all teachers who cannot continue to undergo equal change will gradually become less effective. In practice, few teachers can survive competition from their bright youngsters for longer than 10 years. Shall we employ a faculty to be effective teachers for 10 years and dull old men for 30?

The teacher who gets up in the morning determined to learn something about biological or biosocial systems that he did not know yesterday will have to undergo continual change and therefore he increases his chances of staying in touch with his students. It makes no difference how this drive expresses itself. It may be in the clinic or the laboratory.

Therefore, a departmental chairman selecting a faculty member for a long teaching life chooses one with research experience. Selecting faculty for teaching ability will only make your institution dull.

In the medical center, bright young men interested in a successful professional career will learn a great deal no matter what the teachers do.

Certainly we would be foolish to pay a teacher for what is going to happen without him.

The effectiveness of the teacher must be judged by the things which happen after the student and teacher part company. The immediate communication between student and teacher is usually of more benefit to the teacher than to the student. The interchange causes the teacher to order his thoughts. The movement and rearrangement of material stored in his memory increases the chance for the stored knowledge to be transformed into usable, easily available knowledge and may even evoke an original thought. Usually the student forgets the material unless the contact causes him to undertake intellectual work he would not have done without the student-teacher interaction. The teacher must change his student substrate into its activated form. Most of the ATP required for reaching the activated state must come from the student.

* * * *

Great teachers come from all areas of the medical profession. All have to face one problem: it is impossible to remain the best in an area of medicine for a long period of time. The world belongs to the young, and my resident is tough competition for any professor, part-time or fulltime.[1]

•

The most common error is for the doctor to keep on doing at the age of 50 what he clearly enjoyed at the age of 30. For the majority of teachers, their real excitement wanes after 15 years. They should pass the torch to the youngsters and move on to other areas of responsibilities in the school or community. We should enjoy the young, not compete with them. The young should gain responsibility while they have the drive and enthusiasm to enjoy it. In this way the profession will more effectively mold the lives of men.[1]

•

Research should be carried out with residents and fellows to stimulate their thinking. With older staff, research is a means for keeping minds alert and teaching interesting.[1]

•

The young and the old have different functions. The young are able to give new and more useful information while the older, more wisdom. They can generalize in problem areas from a broader outlook.[1]

* * * *

The Department of Medicine at Duke has been effective in supplying a large number of teachers for other universities. This happy circumstance has come about because we have been able to establish a reasonable number of stable positions with sufficient income to allow the full development of the potential talents. During this period of maturation the faculty member is given enough responsibility in teaching to make him both interested and capable in handling students. When opportunities in other universities open up which represent a potential opportunity for great development, he is both prepared and confident that he is ready for the new opportunity. The VA Hospital has helped us greatly in the final maturation of the young faculty member. There he can operate an area on his own. When the unit is successful, there can be no doubt to whom the credit belongs. Failure is equally obvious.

•

A new medical school curriculum succeeds before it begins, since the faculty has to begin thinking about education again and discussing how they might change their course to make the change. It lends an atmosphere of adventure to the faculty.[1]

* * * *

All members of our department do not have to be alike. We have room for the best clinician, the best teacher and the best scientist, and any possible combinations. We have only one universal requirement: an interest in the University and its teaching program. We do not require a man to be unchanged during his lifetime. He can be the brightest scientist for 10 years, the brightest clinician for 10 years, and the best teacher for 10 years. He remains a man with equal honor in any combination of these capacities.

The University can pay with two commodities: (a) money, and (b) free time. The scientist with free time will be paid less than the clinician who has given up his free time. The scientist will be paid by salary, the clinician will have an unlimited income. The scientist will extract from departmental funds, the clinician will add. Both will teach.

We can markedly modify the direction of a young man's career by the type of financial arrangement. If he is paid a fixed salary and spends an agreed amount of time in practice, he will do no more than the agreement. If he has a colleague who will profit by seeing an additional patient, he has no hesitation in calling his colleague day or night to protect his own free time. Whenever the income increases as the number of patients increase, the net effect is more practice and less free time.

•

Our assistant professors know that they are not tenured; they know that most of them will have to find locations elsewhere. But they know they will have two to five years of growth in an exciting place and that they will have an opportunity to do research and become outstanding teachers.

•

All physicians can have a role in these projections into the future. In our medical center, the fulltime teachers are apt to take the lead—not because they are brighter or more capable, but because they are paid in such a way that they have the leisure time for thinking.

•

The secret of running a successful medical department depends on the chief assembling about him a number of people, any of whom can outdistance him in some field. This also must be done without arousing anxiety and jealousy, if it is to be accomplished.[1]

* * * *

Trained people for giving good medical services in outpatient clinics are not available. Most medical schools run poor outpatient clinics. I suggested to Dr. Davison that the Duke Endowment invest $30,000 yearly in a Duke training program in the medical outpatient clinic. We could give the outpatient the same degree of medical excitement that the hospital has. We would then produce medical personnel oriented to enjoying work in outpatient departments, and a hospital wishing to strengthen its outpatient department could find good professional leadership.

Until effective training programs are organized, attempts to strengthen outpatient departments, including our own, are doomed to failure.

•

Duke-trained people have the great advantage of being equally at home with both public and private patients. They can run a department because they have not been protected by being relieved of administrative chores.

•

In our department a faculty member is either paid a straight salary unrelated to the income he creates or he is paid primarily from the fees from patients whom he sees, and there is no ceiling on income. In the latter instance, he pays his secretary and various assistants. If he is a hard worker, he will use up a considerable amount of our examining space and beds. He will have a considerable income and he will pay a higher departmental tax on that portion of his income beyond $20,000. If he is a slow worker and comes in late and leaves early, he will create little income but use little of our facilities. These arrangements recognize that all men are not equally effective. At certain times of life, one may wish to work harder than at other times. I hope that our department can keep its present flexibility.

* * * *

The Department of Medicine carries the greatest teaching load in the hospital. To teach and remain competitive in the research field, the department must have a clinical staff creating enough funds to stabilize additional members more heavily involved in teaching and research and less involved in practice. The situation is different in Surgery. Because of the greater income created per hour, the surgeons can both practice and do research. Therefore, financing the Department of Surgery is much simpler than financing Medicine.

•

Men in the basic science departments, deans in the medical schools, clinical teachers interested in training doctors for general practice, and university presidents decry the allocation of funds into categorical areas for support of research directly related to a particular disease. They are afraid of the warping forces which can be created in the university structure by vigorous development of various categorical areas. They want to keep clinical research beds equally available for any type of study which may be of interest to the scientist.

•

A clinician in a university hospital works predominantly in one categorical area. He is an expert in cancer, vascular disease, heart disease, arthritis, or diabetes. He faces each day the misery caused by disease. He needs research beds to house his patients and funds to mount as direct an attack on the problem as possible. He has no fears about warping any school or university. He wants to establish sharp cutting edges in his area of patient responsibility and to dispel ignorance which limits his services to his patients. He needs a flow of patients to give a full experience with all the ins and outs of the disease and to keep the urgency of the problems foremost in the minds of himself and his colleagues.

Progress in any university is not made by shoring up the weak areas. It is made by creating areas of excellence which eventually cause other people to attempt to scale the same heights. Outstanding achievement in a categorical area is one way to create an area of excellence.

•

[*Two letters to the American College of Physicians*]: I am enclosing a $15 check for my annual dues. I assume the omission of an academic rate in your schedule is an oversight.

On balance, the contribution of the fulltime faculty to our organization has been greater than the contribution of the organization to the faculty. If necessary, I will pay the $40 fee so that I can voice my opinion. I would not

advise any young fulltime member of my department to join the organization at the rates quoted now. [1–26–62]

[*After further consideration*]: I will enlarge a little on the problem of the
young man in fulltime medicine. The practitioner of internal medicine
usually belongs to the AMA, to the ACP and to some special clinical
society. In addition to these, the man in fulltime medicine must belong to
the Federated Societies and pay dues to the American Physiological Society
or to the society identified with one of the basic science disciplines. He
must take an active part in the societies supporting clinical research, such
as the Society for Clinical Research, the Association of American Physicians,
or the Society for Investigative Dermatology.

His income is not increased by belonging to any of the strictly clinical
societies. His scientific prestige suffers if he does not belong to those
organizations engaged in basic science and clinical research activities. If it
comes to a choice, he will drop his clinical societies.

I do hope this matter will receive a most thoughtful review. [2–5–62]

* * * *

The doctor who reports a case becomes a much better doctor. The doctor
who sits down to answer a question must handle and manipulate ideas to
arrive at a conclusion and, in so doing, has a part in the future.[1]

•

A department of medicine is a place where the demands of the patients
add to the pleasures of the day. The laboratories of the members of a
department of medicine may be indistinguishable from those of the other
scientists in the institution, but the distribution of energy and the satisfactions of the day are different.

•

Education and research are inseparably linked together. Research is the
identification and solution of unsolved problems. Education is the presentation to the student of material which is known and of the problems which
have been solved. Education consists of three steps.

1. the learning of languages, both word language and symbolic languages
which allow the student to explore any area of recorded knowledge;

2. the accumulation and storage of bits of knowledge (memory);

3. the manipulation of these bits of knowledge (thinking).

Research by definition is problem identification and problem solving. It
requires the ability to use the materials and thinking skills given by the
educator in new and original ways.

Education gives man the bits of knowledge and the opportunity to
manipulate the bits. He can engage in problem solving by manipulation of

the bits. If the answers to problems are known, it is not research but an exercise in thinking, involving the correct setting up of logical systems and the proper use of the laboratory. In an educational framework, one can give preliminary research experience by bringing the student to a critical point in history of one discipline. One then gives the student the facts known at that time and the methods of approach to the problem which were then available. The student then has the opportunity to think through the means of solving the problem, using the books available at that time and the laboratory. If he can solve the problem he gains experience in problem solving, in the use of books and in the use of laboratory methods. He encourages his educators to believe that he has research potential. After this stage, the student continues his education by continuing to acquire more language skills, by continuing to gain more bits of information, by continuing active manipulation and rearrangement of the bits and, in addition, he is given time and facilities to attack unsolved problems which he has identified as both important and solvable. Once the problem is solved, new bits of knowledge are now available for use in the education of the student in the area. Thus the frontier of education is in the laboratory.

In any educational institution the primary product is molded and trained manpower. The man capable of reading books written in many languages, the man experienced in manipulation of these bits, and the man capable of using this background for the identification and solution of now-solvable problems is the most important product of the educational system. Only when this product continues to engage in education and research can he reproduce his kind. Thus advanced education and research become inseparable.

The educated man engaged in research can and does operate over a wide spectrum of activities. He can remain in a university and reproduce himself by investing a large amount of time in the education of students. In this frame of reference his own research is one of the methods used in advanced education, and the new knowledge created is incidental to the main product: trained manpower. He may elect to go into a research institute sponsored by foundations, industry or government where he will engage primarily in research. He will always be teaching some of the already-trained people in his laboratory, but his primary product will be new knowledge rather that trained manpower.

In the engineering field the social system has developed which allows the educated man to flow back and forth between university, the research institute, and facilities for production which convert the knowledge gained from research into products useful for people. We need to improve our social system in the health area to the point where there is a freer interchange between research and the use of research knowledge. This will require new methods of financing and accounting. The many products of space technology now flowing in normal economic channels were developed by a large investment of funds in products which were not purchasable by individuals in the community. Similar investments in production of systems and methods to use the research will have to be made before the products of the research in the health fields are readily purchasable by the individual. The universities, hospitals, and industry cannot ignore this challenge.

•

The medical school of a generation ago had many of the characteristics of a small college. Its student body was kept relatively homogeneous by rigid admission requirements. The school attempted to transmit to the student a well-defined body of knowledge in both preclinical and clinical areas. It anticipated that most students would have a limited graduate experience and that the school must cover all the facts necessary for the practice of medicine. At graduation, the product was relatively homogeneous and, in general, each graduate could be replaced by any other graduate. The amount of elective work allowed was small because granting elective time meant leaving out material considered essential by the faculty.

The faculty was small and time to devote to research was limited. The entire effort was directed toward the undergraduate student, and the worth of a faculty member was gauged by his teaching effort. A large investment of faculty time was made to bring along the slower students. The faculty itself was not highly specialized. The reward system emphasized teaching over scholarship.

When a college grows into a university, many changes occur. Students are less homogeneous at entry. They come from wider geographical and cultural backgrounds, and they arrive on the campus at widely different stages of training. The advanced graduate students appear in ever-increasing number, and kudos among the faculty are handed out more and more often for scholarship rather than for teaching of undergraduate students. Those students who are slower to mature and who need more individual attention become fewer in number as, gradually, they select smaller, less complex schools.

The faculty of the emerging university becomes increasingly specialized and is willing to accept earlier specialization among the students. The amount of required work is decreased. The faculty, actively engaged in research itself, appreciate the role of research as an educational tool. Students in various honors courses have the opportunity to engage in research as a part of their education. As the number of students spending more than four calendar years in the institution is large, the division between graduate and undergraduate work becomes less rigid. More emphasis is placed on the teaching of mathematics, physics, chemistry, electronics, sociology and psychology as a series of languages, because increasing numbers of students will need to read books written in these symbols.

As these changes in philosophy and practice occur in the educational system, stresses appear in the college social system. The older faculty members feel that there is too much emphasis on research and that too many young staff members teach the introductory undergraduate courses. Moreover, the older members of the college community are sometimes reluctant to give equal status to the increased administrative personnel needed to operate these complex and expensive research ventures. Academic rank becomes less important as the more complex university gives a wider range of rewards.

In the last 20 years, many forces have been at work which have affected the medical scene and produced changes in medical schools. Many of these changes paralleled those which occur with the growth of a college into a university.

. . . The medical schools did not want to narrow their intake. Their role was to supply manpower for the whole health field. The non-scientist who wishes to give service to his fellow man will treat many more sick persons than the quantitative biologist who is interested in how man functions in health and disease. Conversely, the scientist will serve few patients with his own hands, but he will create new knowledge which will increase greatly the effectiveness of the practicing doctor.

The solution in most schools has been to use the four medical school years for a general survey of the medical field. This solution allows all of the medical students to have a common experience regardless of their preparation, but it produces no student who has really mastered any one discipline. The internship is one year more of general experience. Then come two years in the service and one more year of refresher work before the candidate decides to specialize in a clinical area. He still has time to learn what the current specialist does in clinical practice, but he has spent too much time in general areas to master one or more of the scientific disciplines which allow him to make a major contribution in his field of special interest. His trouble cannot be that he has not put in enough years. He has spent four years in college, surveying; four years in medical school, surveying; and four years in hospitals and the service, surveying. Unfortunately, by the time the surveying is over, he may be too old to learn.

The health professions are certain to become the largest users of trained manpower in the world. Because of the demands of the people, money will continue to come into this area more easily than into many other fields. Universities and medical schools have not wished to face the tremendous demand for trained manpower in the health field, nor have they realized their inability to meet this tide with their present facilities. Properly used, this surge offers a great challenge for university development. The day will pass when university presidents are pitied for the headaches posed by their health areas. Instead, they will be envied for the opportunities for general university development opened up by their medical centers.[4]

•

Our prime product is not the care of patients or the production of new knowledge by research. Men are our prime product: men to care for sick and well patients, men to do medical research, men to carry out the varied functions needed by the health field.[1]

* * * *

For the production of the manpower we do use both tools of research and the tools of medical care and its implementation. I would point out to you that the educational field is of necessity inefficient. You can never educate anybody to think if you are at the same time requiring him to have maximal efficiency in the use of those things which he has already learned. Education is essentially a time in which you put bits of information into people's heads and then you give them the opportunity and the chance to move them around to build new structures, to make new things and, above all things, to make mistakes.

So, an educational institution by its very nature is an inefficient institution. In the clinical training of manpower, it has to remain in part inefficient in regard to even the use of technical, secretarial and other kinds of help, for the very real reason that you don't want to raise the basic cost of the unit in which the physician is getting his education to the point where it has to produce the maximal amount of services. If it does, you cannot carry out the education.

* * * *

[*Veteran's Administration Hospitals*]: The Dean's Committee hospitals have worked excellently when the hospital and the university have been able to identify a number of areas where the sum of the activities of the school and the VA hospital working together has been greater than the sum of their activities working apart. Mutual needs and achievements bind units closely together. Over a long run, the VA hospital will not invest the time necessary for integration with a university program unless tangible results occur. Similarly, members of the senior faculty of the university will not devote time to the Dean's Committee hospital unless by so doing they can more nearly meet university aims.

•

Reasons for research in the Veterans Administration are:

1. to give the practicing physician better answers to health problems of the veterans;

2. to focus research efforts on those diseases which are most common in the veteran population;

3. to use the facilities of VA hospitals for cooperative clinical studies which will benefit both the veteran and the non-veteran;

4. to insure the veteran that he is being cared for by physicians of curiosity and imagination who will bring the recent advances in science to the care of the sick;

5. to enable the university-affiliated VA hospital to give clinical training to students, interns and residents equal to that given in other portions of the university medical center; and

6. to train basic scientists and physician-scientists. The VA is a major user of trained manpower. There is not enough manpower to go around, and the VA must be a producer of trained manpower as well as a user.

The VA must engage in research at both the clinical and basic science levels. Without basic research, there will be few useful answers to most of our unsolved problems. Without active basic science laboratories, advanced training for the physician-scientist will be inadequate. Without clinical research, the problems of the sick will never impinge on the basic scientist. Without clinical research, the advances in basic science will not be translated into better patient care.

Funds should flow from Congress to VA and Congress to NIH to VA. In practice, most of the funds from the NIH will flow into university-affiliated hospitals. The VA will have to accept the reality that all its hospitals will not have productive research programs. Those without active research programs will be users of trained manpower and will contribute relatively little to the trained manpower pool.

The stable yearly appropriation from Congress to VA will allow it to recruit men on a career basis. The NIH funds are available to allow growth of the program in competition with other programs. If the VA-sponsored scientists cannot competitively win approval of their research programs through NIH mechanisms, then the VA is spending its own funds unwisely. The stable recurrent appropriation to the VA and the competitively sought NIH funds give the VA system the same type of financing which is present in other parts of the university. The university supplies a floor but the ceiling is defined competitively.

No institution giving complete medical care can carry out its program without personnel and space for research. Complicated clinical care too quickly enters into areas of the unknown. There must be an area of the service where the physicians and scientists are less pressed by the giving of immediate medical care. These men must have a large hand in the design of medical care for tomorrow. Every university-affiliated VA hospital needs two types of research space:

1. that immediately contiguous to wards where unsolved clinical problems are studied, and
2. a laboratory research building where physician-scientists work and basic scientists work. The absence of a well-designed research space has handicapped the VA in its recruiting program and is having a progressively unfavorable effect on the program of medical care.

•

We run a completely integrated service with students, interns and residents. The VA is staffed in Medicine entirely by men of my own selection. It provides an ideal opportunity to tell whether a young man can run his own show. We have no permanent staff at the VA. Either the man succeeds and climbs the academic ladder or he goes into practice. This reopens the slot for the next bright man.

I determine when a member of our faculty moves into the VA and when he moves out.

In times of shortage of personnel, the two hospitals are treated equally.

We have a larger staff at the VA than their table of organization calls for. This allows us to maintain an active research program and take care of the patients. We have enlarged the staff by the use of outside funds and by the use of special VA funds. In other words, geography does not automatically determine the source of support.

Professional decisions and research projects are determined by the Department of Medicine rather than by the manager or chief of professional services. I back up completely the professional independence of my faculty. I determine whether areas of assignment of interns and residents are of teaching value. If they are not of teaching value, the assignments are not made.

I have carefully delineated our areas of mutual interest with the VA and have made no attempt to milk the VA. In our areas of mutual interest I have taken complete responsibility for professional staffing.

I operate with a small budget, but one in which there is little waste. If a man earns an appreciable portion of his income by practice, we pay him $2,500 from our budget. He makes the rest by practice, pays for his own office help and contributes to our departmental fund. There is no limit on his income, and we keep our departmental tax low enough to make it profitable for him to see an additional patient.

If a man creates only a minor portion of his income by practice, he contributes an agreed-upon amount of time to practice, but he profits none by extending the time. He has no qualms of conscience in referring patients to colleagues who will profit financially by the referral. The more the faculty member lives like a preclinical colleague, the closer his salary approaches the established local salary scale of the preclinical faculty. The common habit of paying one-half the salary, making the rest in practice with a fixed ceiling, is the surest way to waste the university budget.

We have a flexible social system which allows for change. We recognize many forms of excellence. We have not tied income to the academic ladder....

The system is . . . in part self-selecting. There being a very limited amount of hard money, everyone knows that he has to create something with a marketable value: research, patient care, teaching, administration. Because there is no papa to turn to, initiative can be taken at many levels. We don't give much, but we don't have many rules. [1966]

•

There are service assignments in the VA which are too service-oriented for the best training. The admitting office area is a good example. In most instances, a conscientious Dean's Committee will insist that this be a salaried position not related to training.

* * * *

Our problem relates to the fact that stimulation of one area in the health field led to immediate shortages in others. This was to be expected in the health field and its related sciences where chronic undernourishment had existed for a long time. Fifteen years ago, research positions in biological sciences were unknown in most universities and hospitals. Research workers were produced in small numbers because a larger group would have starved. We trained no medical scientists because there was no way for them to eat. [1965]

•

The man responsible for clinical research in the future should have had a rich research experience involving some area of quantitative biology.

•

An appreciation of the importance of basic science training and of the importance of physicists, engineers, biochemists, geneticists, mathematicians, psychologists, and other scientists in solving problems of biology was hastened by the development of the intramural program of the National

Institutes of Health. Many of the brightest young men with M.D. degrees spent their two years of service time in this intramural program. For this two-year period, the customary rapid postgraduation movement to ever-increasing clinical responsibility was broken. Many of these men had a type of experience which they would never have selected voluntarily, because it was outside the cultural pattern of the usual M.D. program. But, being bright and accustomed to hard work, they rapidly adapted to their new role as scientists. When they returned to the medical schools, many as faculty members, they brought with them a different notion of the role of the non-medical scientists in the medical world. Coming up against career research men, they had gained an appreciation for the need of a good knowledge of scientific language as a prerequisite for a career in which they expected support from the research dollar.

•

I can see the problem of a granting agency which has no real way of separating the sheep from the goats. Is the residency training being used as a means to prepare for practice in the usual sense, or is it being used for intellectual development and to enlarge research opportunities? Clearly, most residencies serve as preparation for practice. The chance of making mistakes frightens the fellowship granting boards.

•

During the holidays, I have had time to reflect on the impact of present NIH programs and projected NIH programs on the training of future leaders in clinical medicine. Some of these men will be in academic medicine and some of them will be the leading physicians and surgeons in their communities but, together, they will provide leadership in medical affairs.

Traineeships set up under the categorical institutes by their very nature invite specialization at an early stage and, for people content to work in a narrow area, this may be desirable. For leaders in broader areas, one needs approximately three years of general training in clinical medicine before moving into the areas of categorical interests. At present, these three years have to be financed by the intern and resident or by his family. By forgoing this general training, he can more easily become self-supporting through the categorical institutes.

I do not believe that the categorical institutes should give up these efforts to attract men into their areas of interest, but I do think that funds should be available for support of men who want the basic training in the broad areas before specialization. My own inclination would be to have all general training in medicine and surgery supported by the Health Council. Categorical support could come in early if it best suited the development of the man, or it could follow after the first three more basic years.

I do not see any end to this except for fairly general support of residency training. Before the War there were very few programs which gave more than three years of training. Many of these have been extended to five years, the two additional years being supported by the categorical institutes. Unless some more solid support is given to the first years of general training, financial pressure will force more and more men to move prematurely into the categorical areas.

•

We forget that, prior to 15 years ago, a man devoting a large part of his time to research in these areas would have had no source of income. He could create a livelihood by seeing sick patients in these special areas of disease and by this mechanism the specialists in these areas were created. They became expert in the handling of one or another area of illness in the light of known knowledge, and they learned a great deal from the sick patients. Neither by training nor by the distribution of their time were these men able to bring to bear on their problems the modern tools of biophysics, biochemistry, genetics, electronics, or engineering.

•

In the last 15 years, careers in research have been opened by the volunteer health agencies and by the National Institutes of Health. The universities have enlarged their faculties and the Markle Program, under Mr. John Russell's direction, has been most helpful at the university level. Mr. Russell early appreciated that the universities (the place for identifying and growing brains) had to be strengthened to supply the increased need for trained personnel. He knew that the university had to produce, in addition to the usual M.D., a great variety of medical scientists and he early appreciated that the use of the university talent for project research (immediate answer to a current problem) might stop the production of new scientists. [1963]

* * * *

There is no doubt that we could recruit, educate and license general practitioners. The question at issue is: will they fit into the buying habits of the American public? Everyone has seen the customers bypass the general country store for the suburban supermarket. Will the generalist be obsolete 20 years from now as people go towards increasing dependence on specialization? We have a large quantity of unemployed aerospace engineers today. Will we have an equally large number of unemployed general physicians tomorrow?

•

The health field finds itself at the crossroads. It must either strengthen its educational program or fail in its mission to supply personnel to give health services to the nation and to staff the research laboratories of the future.

Fifteen years ago the educational service and research capabilities of the nation resided in the same people. Funds not being available to support a person devoting full time to research, he made a portion of his living by teaching, by giving health services and by assuming administrative duties within the health area or university. We are now well into the development of a new generation who have been supported by research funds throughout their training and who now are receiving career appointments to remain in the research field. These men have little experience in giving health care, little responsibility for the training of men who will succeed them, and little experience with administrative matters outside their own laboratories. They are the producers of new knowledge rather than of men.

The program of supporting research and research training has been an outstanding success. For the first time, both the government and universities have accepted the responsibility for establishing research careers on a large scale. We realize that we are developing only one-prong research of a three-prong responsibility: namely, research, health care and teaching. Nevertheless, a start had to be made somewhere and there would clearly be some overflow from the research area into the two other areas of responsibility. This has occurred and, at present, all three areas are improved.

Our problem is that the old pattern is breaking down. One has to only look at the shining new research facilities and the outdated medical school teaching and university hospital facilities to grasp the imbalance in the present situation. Capable faculty prefer quarters and appointments in the research area and avoid assuming the old responsibilities of health care and teaching and administration. Many investigators do their best research at an early age. Biological changes occur which may prevent the investigator from entering new fields and bring his productive work to a halt. In former years, these men moved from research into teaching. With the current scarcity of teaching funds and the many men financed by research mechanisms, such an orderly transition from one function to another is prevented. The health field is the one area of endeavor where one would expect its leaders to appreciate the reality of steady biological change. It is unrealistic to expect the man of 55 to be the same person he was at 35.

We must either decrease our research drive and development or strengthen the basic educational facilities and staff who create service, educational and research personnel. Knowing full well the number of unsolved problems in the health field, it is obviously better judgment to restore balance to our program by increasing support in the educational and health service fields than by decreasing the rate of growth of the research program.

We have always known that the present research support mechanisms of the National Institutes of Health are not intended to solve the educational problems in the health field. In spite of this limitation, medical educators have given full support to the development of research support. The time has now come for the leaders in the research field to give as generously of their time and effort to help obtain the needed funds and facilities to provide the basic education for health personnel who can staff the areas of health service, education and research. Unless these capable leaders of research appreciate the present situation and put their best efforts into increasing the basic educational program in the medical schools, they will sharply curtail the future development of their research goal.

We need to ask the leaders in the research area to sponsor the development of the entire health area or we must develop new leaders. We believe Senator Hill and Representative Fogarty have the vision to spearhead the entire program. If they do not, new leadership must be sought. It is logical to use the same supporters and leaders who have spearheaded the research effort, because their stake can be protected only by moving forward in the other areas. But move we must; if necessary, without the leadership of the men who have developed research support.

The immediate educational needs in the health field are: 1) predoctoral support of medical students; 2) increase in teaching facilities in all areas supporting the health field: This includes medical and nursing school buildings and teaching hospitals; 3) support of graduate medical and nursing students; 4) support of university faculty and paramedical personnel when not engaged in research; and 5) increase in number of students of nursing, medical and paramedical disciplines.

* * * *

The American people and its government are becoming progressively involved with the proper use of the "health dollar". The health dollar must provide for 1) education of health professionals, 2) delivery of health care, and 3) research at both the basic and applied levels. Public policy in the health field can be made by an informed electorate. Each person has some interest in health, the issues can be described in non-technical terms, and there are no security reasons for holding back information.

The public needs to know the consequences of expanding or restricting the health dollar in any of these areas.

There is at present a great deal of emphasis on restricting research, decreasing the scientific component of our educational programs, and expanding our systems for delivering health care.

The public needs to know about the basic difference between an effective program for delivery of health care (the medicine of today) and the development of programs which remove the problem (research and the medicine of tomorrow). The differences in these two approaches can be told in very graphic terms. We can try, and are trying, to devise better systems to care for the people now suffering from congenital defects produced by rubella. This can be contrasted with the elimination of this problem by vaccination.

The educational lead time for bioscience and for better information systems leading to improved care is long. False steps today can lead to paralysis tomorrow.

Medicaid is a striking example of the passage of a law without adequate information being available to the Congress or Executive branch. In the absence of a uniform federal-state system of data gathering, there was no possible way to estimate the actual impact and cost of this legislation on health care. This legislation was proposed and passed by the Congress. They had to pass it or not pass it. No mechanism existed to field test in advance any of the component parts.

There are already a great many laws affecting the health field, and each year there will be more. Doctors out in the field are aware of the problems created by these laws and by the operating agencies produced by them. Once the laws are put into operation, they gain support at the agency level. The new agencies, and the personnel employed by them, become part of the large governmental bureaucracy. Regardless of the absurdities which develop, or the lack of progress in achieving the goals which the lawmakers envisaged, the new agencies will not disappear.

Anyone who has tried to develop a sensible building program in a medical center involving facilities for education, ambulatory patients, bed patients, animals, research, library, and the community becomes aware of the fragmentation of health funds among governmental agencies and the inability of any one area in government to coordinate all the many avenues for support to achieve the overall objectives for which the lawmakers think they passed the laws. Even more discouragement will occur if one attempts to instigate new programs which involve a marriage between agencies supporting welfare, vocational training, education, new careers and health care for the disabled and the aged. You will find many statements of good will but no real help.

The time has come for the Congress to address itself to ways and means of testing legislation by appropriate studies before it enacts legislation which will have an unpredictable effect on our nation. We need a program of research to study the mechanisms for constructing laws which will more nearly achieve the goals for which they are designed.

My suggestion would be to make funds available to the major committees of the Congress for initiation of pilot projects before passing legislation which will affect the entire country. The laws as now passed frequently allow for demonstration projects under the new public laws. The law may be so constructed that the demonstration project must operate within very narrow confines, because the overlapping and functionally related areas were not identified in the legislation. A demonstration project before the passage of final legislation would seem to be a better approach.

Further study may show that my proposal for approaching this difficult problem is unwise and that there is a better way to solve the problem. The proposal is not made to defend but, rather, as a means of drawing attention to the serious need for research and experimentation to improve mechanisms for designing legislation. [1972]

References

1. Schoonmaker F, Metz, E. Just Say For Me. World Press Inc., Denver, 1968.
2. Stead EA. Ann. Int. Med. 72: 271, 1970.
3. Stead EA. Pharos of AOA 32: 54, 1969.
4. Stead EA. J. Med. Educ. 39: 368, 1964.

5

Most Medical Problems Are Not Curable

THE CHALLENGE OF MEDICAL PRACTICE

Most medical problems are not curable. They represent the interaction between the patient and his environment. Once the patient is out of his usual environment, he will begin to mend. In the course of his stay in the hospital, a number of studies will be carried out to understand why the particular patient does poorly in his environment. Sometimes the studies are helpful, but the emotional support of the hospital personnel and the break in organism-environmental relationship is more often helpful.

•

The worse the disease the more useless the doctor.

•

A doctor often cannot solve the problem or cure a patient. Therefore, he, along with the patient, must learn to live with it.

•

When I see a patient come into the hospital in congestive heart failure over and over, I look on it as failure of the house staff to realize that there is some disease that can't be handled.[1]

•

If one doesn't know what is actually going on, then one doesn't really know how to handle it.

•

The best advice you can give a young man with coronary artery disease is not to invest all his resources in medical care. We have so little to offer.

•

I would rather be called to see someone who is frightened than to see someone who is dying. The results of treating the first are obviously so much better.[1]

•

I have always been interested in self-limited illnesses of unknown etiology. These illnesses have a definite time of onset, run a widely variable course and end in complete recovery. During the course of the illness the patient needs the type of protection afforded any ill patient but, when the illness is over, the patient is well and requires no further protection. The fact that the illness is self-limited is frequently masked by treatment. For this reason the frequency of this syndrome in practice is hard to determine.

The quickest way to become knowledgeable in this area is to take complete health histories in a large number of patients. The periods when the patient was out of work more than one week or when he visited a doctor more than three times in a month are recorded. In this type of survey, the diagnosis is commonly not helpful because usually it is made more from desperation than from knowledge. Of much more importance is the account of what happened. How did the patient feel? What complaints were present? What did the doctor do? What special examinations were made? What treatment was instigated? What did the wife say? How did the mother and mother-in-law react? What was the pattern of recovery? What was the total cost of the illness?

Many diseases which are usually self-limited have a known etiology and well-defined pathology. Infectious hepatitis is a good example. Some are of unknown etiology but have a well enough defined clinical course and pathologic findings to allow definitive subgrouping to which a diagnostic term can be given. Infectious mononucleosis is a good example of this group. The physician is comfortable in the treatment of these well-defined types of self-limited illness. He is less certain when the laboratory tests are normal and when the illness extends beyond a week.

Many self-limited illnesses begin with fatigue, loss of libido and evidence of either irritability or lack of inhibition in the nervous system. Because of the absence of any laboratory tests for illness, the doctor frequently wonders if the patient is ill. The patient is, of course, the smarter. He *knows* that he is ill! The patient frequently becomes desperate because he feels that if the doctor doesn't do something he will become steadily worse. The doctor with experience knows that the patient was well until a given time, has been sick until the present, and will eventually be well again. He knows that he must devise a way for the patient to live until recovery occurs but that this will occur without his help. The doctor's role is to support the patient, to prevent him from making unwise decisions about his future and to avoid the development of patterns of behavior that will handicap the patient when he is well.

These episodes of self-limited illness in productive persons must be separated from experiences with patients who are chronic complainers and who have a lifetime pattern of difficulty in performing. I do not know how to draw the line between some of these episodes of self-circumscribed illness and the disease syndrome that we call depression. Both occur in productive people and both end in recovery. The wide clinical spectrum of the self-circumscribed illnesses makes it very unlikely that they can have a single etiology.

The doctor who sees the patient in the first days and weeks of such self-limited illness has the most difficult time. He doesn't know whether his patient will be alive or dead four weeks later. The doctor who sees the patient later has a tremendous advantage. He can eliminate all diseases which would have given definitive findings in a period of time equal to that between onset and the present. Interestingly enough, in the medical center we often see these patients after recovery begins. The clinical improvement rarely goes smoothly. One or more downturns on a generally rising curve is common. Both doctor and patient become discouraged with these downswings, and referral at this point is common.

Patients are frequently apologetic for using your time when they discover that they are getting well without any definite therapy. I have always enjoyed caring for these patients. What gives a doctor any more satisfaction than a well patient? Even if God did the curing, I kept the devil away during the period of despair![2]

* * * *

The patient can always produce more phenomena than I can ever explain.

•

Some doctors believe there is an explanation for everything, but most biologic phenomena I see I don't know the explanation for.

•

Because every biological system is different from every other one and because every observer brings some bias to the scene it is easier to learn incorrectly than correctly from the practice of medicine.

•

The older doctor does practice differently from the younger person. Patients grow old with their doctor and they are frequently happier with his old-fashioned ways than they are with the modern services rendered by the young man.

•

I have nothing against being somewhat a quack. I always have been a quack. The problem is that medicine doesn't lend itself to being overly scientific.

•

A doctor who believes that anticoagulants neither help nor harm his patient can carry out a randomized study. A doctor who believes, on the basis of his clinical experience, that anticoagulants are useful cannot ethically participate in the study. Neither can a doctor who believes they are harmful.

Many doctors know that certain things are useful or harmful before they are ascertained statistically. I certainly know, from my experiences as a doctor, that smoking effects the respiratory tree adversely. It would not have been ethical for me to have randomized patients into smoking and non-smoking populations.

•

God takes care of the physician.

* * * *

Many people who have no demonstrable illness have many complaints. The fit between the well body and the use of the well body may be poor. When the integration between the body and the environment is poor, dysfunction occurs and complaining appears. We can think of an analogy with machines. A tractor plowing a field is a fine instrument; as a racing car, it is a complete flop. Each of us is a particular instrument and, when given our best fit, we perform well. Given a poor fit, our bodies complain and we go to the doctor.

A part of your role will be to listen to the patient, to learn the peculiarities of his brain and to devise the best fit between his biological machine and the uses to which he puts it. Most of the cues will not come from conventional testing. They will come from an analysis of his reactions to other people and from an honest separation of the things that actually give him satisfaction from those things that would have given satisfaction to some ideal person that he admired in his youth. He rarely turns out to be that ideal person, so his satisfactions may come in very different ways.

Confronted with these difficult problems, the body complains to the brain, and the person goes in search of a healer. He may turn to the practitioners of scientific medicine but, if relief is not found (and it rarely will be if the doctor practices only as a scientist), he will turn to a variety of non-scientific healers: Christian Scientists, homeopaths, chiropractors, yogis, acupuncturists, meditationalists, astrologers and palmists. What should be your attitude towards these other healers?

The scientifically trained doctor has two advantages over the other healers. He knows how to use science when it is helpful in healing, and he knows that both he and a great variety of healers can make the patient perform better without altering the structure of any portion of the body except the brain. A person incapacitated by coronary arterial disease may, by the proper use of art, go back to full activity. The scientific doctor knows that this does not mean that the coronary arteries have changed. If a yogi produced the same good clinical result, he would think that he had changed the coronary arteries. He would not appreciate that the change was limited to the brain.

In time, as the behavior of the brain is understood, science will replace art. Until that time arrives, we should respect and help our nonscientific healers because, in a large part of our daily practice, we are using various nonscientific methods just as they do.

•

The modern doctor is able to tell when scientific medicine can be useful. This is true for only the minority of problems brought to us by our patients. If science at its present stage of development is unable to benefit the patient, we should not deny him access to other healers operating on a mystical base. The mystical operator will never understand science, and he will always believe that he has changed the disease process when his patient improves. He cannot understand that a symptom may disappear because of a reversible alteration of the nervous system without any change in the disease process originally responsible for the symptom. He believes that the disappearance of the angina is equivalent to eliminating the coronary arterial disease.

The best way to handle the problem would be to have a department store for sick patients. At the door would be the scientific doctor. If he understands the problem and can bring science to bear on it, he would treat the patient. If he did not understand the problem but knew that science had nothing to offer, he would allow the patient to enter the store. Healers of all types would display their wares, and the patient could choose that health artist who most appealed to him. This approach would satisfy many patients who are unhappy with the present system.

•

Doctors are trained to maximize the performance of persons during the longest possible period of time. They identify the existing structure of the body at any one point in time and, on the basis of their knowledge, advise the person how best to handle his body to obtain maximal performance at minimal discomfort. In order to perform this function, the physician must divide people into various subgroups. The more precise the subgrouping, the more relevant is the advice of the physician.

A small amount of general advice is useful to the population at large and can be given without the physician's becoming involved in subgrouping. For example, all people should avoid the guillotine because it severs the head of those in all subgroups; bullets piercing the brain stem kill all persons; falls above a certain height are always fatal.[3]

We have normal values for many body functions. The ranges of normal values are always large because all regulation is dependent upon any particular function moving far enough from its average value to set in motion mechanisms to return it toward the baseline.[1]

Any measurements of the normal can't be applied to the sick.

It's hard separating functional and organic because both produce anatomical changes. We are what we are because of structure.[1]

* * * *

[*An internist looks at behavior*]: The theme of this discussion is that all behavior is determined by structure. Changes in the structure are most easily demonstrated by functional tests. By using two kinds of tests, one can determine if an automobile engine will run: 1) he can examine atom by atom the structure of the car, and 2) he can turn on the ignition key, step on the starter, and quickly know if the anatomy of the motor allows it to run. All of us would elect to use the functional method of testing to evaluate the structure of the motor.

When I refer to structure, I am including ultramicroscopic arrangement of matter as well as the microscopic and gross aspects of structure. For the purposes of this discussion, the change of glucose to glycogen, the change in adenosine triphosphate to adenosine diphosphate, the change in hemoglobin to bilirubin are treated as changes in structure. The movement of hydrocortisone from the adrenal gland to the blood represents a change in structure. The depolarization of muscle cell or of a nerve cell again is accomplished by a change in structure.

Physicians take histories, do physical examinations, and perform laboratory tests in an attempt to characterize the individual patient. They then group patients with similar characteristics into subgroups. By knowing the natural history of the subgroup, they try to devise means by which the members of the subgroup can have a more favorable prognosis than the subgroup normally has in the absence of medical care.

The physician uses a familiar frame of reference in determining whether his patient is similar to or different from other patients. If the patient says that he has uncontrollable bleeding when the skin is cut or a tooth is pulled, the physician says he is different from people who bleed little with these kinds of trauma. If the doctor finds an apical diastolic murmur with a presystolic accentuation, he knows that this patient is different from people without this murmur. If he finds that the red blood cells sickle when their oxygen tension falls, he again assigns this patient to a particular subgroup.

Differences in people are made more obvious by extending the methods of examination. For example, two pieces of painted wood may appear, on casual examination, to be identical. On driving a nail into each piece, it is obvious that one is much harder than the other. Extending the testing has revealed dissimilarity. It is clear that, since the woods differ, one will be more useful in certain situations than will the other. The physician may select 100 males of age 40 years who seem to have identical hearts when examined at rest. The dissimilarity of these hearts is easily established by observing the wide range of adaptation to the stress of hypertension or an arteriovenous communication.

The chemist, of course, uses similar methods to establish identity or nonidentity. He compares two proteins which can hydrolyze substrates; he examines their color, their solubility in different solvents, their isoelectric point, their light-diffusing properties, their behavior in the ultracentrifuge, their behavior in an electrical field, and the effects of different environmental changes in viscosity. If all these stresses give the same value for both proteins, he is tempted to say that they are the same protein. But he knows that further testing for substrate specificity, for example, may show that identity is not present.

The physician proceeds in the same way. He knows that his patient at any given point in time is a unique organism and that similarities between the patient and other persons or groups of persons have to be determined by appropriate testing. He knows that at any one moment the biological organism (the patient) has a definitive structure which is the result of genetic information modified by environmental input and that, at any one point in time, the potential response of the organism is tightly tied to this structure. Just as the chemist wants to know the source of his protein, be it mollusk muscle or bat wing, so that doctor wants to know the source of his organism, and the genetic and environmental background of his patient. The doctor knows that some genotypes are particularly sensitive to environmental influences (lack of tanning in pituitary insufficiency). The taking of the family history and the developmental history of the patient and his siblings is an exciting adventure. The patient will have more similarities to some members of his family or to some combination of those members than he will to the population at large.

The next step in history taking is to note the influence of environment on the development of the organism. In taking this part of the history, one will watch particularly two aspects of the problem: 1) he will define those environmental factors which are or have been of importance in modifying either reversibly or irreversibly the structural characteristics of the organism, and 2) he will define existing structural characteristics of the organism at any given time by the observed response to stimuli. Although both these factors—namely, the alteration of structure in a reversible or irreversible way and the demonstration of the structure of the organism at any one instance by the response to an environmental stimulus—are operative together, the relative importance of each factor may vary greatly.

When thalidomide is given at a critical time during the development of the fetus, major congenital anomalies result. At other times, the drug is without demonstrated harmful effects. Experience teaches that certain environmental stimuli are relatively inert when the organism has one structure, and may be very active when the organism has another structure. The imprinting of the baby chick of a duck as its mother when the exposure of the chick to the duck is appropriately timed is an example of a structural change easily induced on one structure (baby chick) and which will not work with another structure (a similar chick a few days older). The effects of environmental stimuli, therefore, are frequently time-dependent because the structure of the organism is continually changing with time. Reversible changes in structure may be part of usual biological development or they may be dependent on acquired abnormalities. A 20-year old man may have a large intake of salt without any weight gain. During a period of acute nephritis, he will have a large gain in weight and may drown on this high salt intake. After recovery, he may again eat the same amount of salt without swelling.

In the physical examination, the physician again looks for differences which allow subgrouping. If he is a wise physician, he increases the likelihood of finding differences by observing the response of the body to emotional and physical stresses. He finds bradycardia in two patients. One heart responds to exercise with an increase in heart rate; the other heart does not increase its rate. He knows that his test of the behavior of the heart with exercise has defined certain morphological differences in the hearts of the two men.

In the laboratory, we use the same frame of reference. Identical urine specimens give identical values. Nonidentical urine specimens give different values. X-ray examinations, pathological examinations, serologic examinations, bacteriologic examinations are used in this same context.

The physician becomes increasingly aware of reversible changes in structure which are brought out by appropriate testing. He knows that the eosinophil count taken before activity begins in the morning will be different than the count in mid-morning. He does not expect the patient to have the same structure in mid-morning as in the early morning. He knows that a carbon dioxide tension, normally present in sleep from decreased ventilation, would cause an increased ventilation in an awake person. This is one of the many behavioral differences that let him know that the sleeping person has different structure from a person who is awake. The physician knows that a person receiving a second load of glucose two hours after an initial load will have a different response from that observed after the first glucose. He knows the patient has a different structure after the first load and that it can be documented by change in behavior to the second stimulus.

A man walks up two flights of stairs. He has a different structure at the top of the stairs than he had at the bottom. Again, the difference is defined by a different response to the same stimulus.

The physician then begins his examination with two pieces of general information: 1) the patient is unlike any other patient he has ever cared for, and 2) the patient is undergoing continual change from millisecond to millisecond. He has to evaluate the quantitative aspects of the differences, and he has to make up his mind as to how important is the rate of change. In a normal-acting 20-year old man, the rate of change may be so low that the doctor will do no more than note the changes which have occurred at intervals from one to five years. In a patient with an acute myocardial infarct, the rate of change may be sufficiently great to require continuous electronic monitoring. The structural changes which occur will be manifested in changes in behavior.

As years go by, the patient will give information indicating that the environment has a different effect than it used to have; the physical examination will show changes in the skin, the lens of the eye, the lung and blood vessels, and laboratory findings and x-ray studies will show change. Whenever the fit between the current state of the organism and the requirements of its environment is poor, the patient will be symptomatic. The development of symptoms indicates either that the unchanged system is now heavily loaded and therefore functions less effectively, or that the system itself has undergone changes which are first demonstrated by a decrease in performance under an unchanged load. Either change will make the load of living seem greater but in the second instance the load is really not greater but, rather, the machine is less capable of carrying the load. In clinical practice, both situations may occur singly or together. In the practice of internal medicine, a change in the machine as the initiating factor is seen more frequently than a change in the load. Once the system begins to operate poorly, with the usual development of family repercussions, economic problems attendant to medical care, the altered feeling states of the patient and those whom he touches during the day, secondary increase in load is common.

Many reversible changes in structure may cause the same loads to be heavier or lighter. Physical changes in the body produced by the monthly pituitary-ovarian cycle are well known to us all. Recurrent cyclic changes occurring during each 24-hour period are common in human beings. Periods of elation and depression occur in us all and are manifestations of changes in structure. The autonomic instability and fatigue caused by many illnesses occur in varying degrees in the population.

The physician knows that all purposeful behavior which he observes in patients is channelled through the nervous system. He knows that the structure of this portion of the organism is subject to the same interplay of genetic and environmental influences which characterize all portions of the biological system. He knows that there are many central nervous systems in the same organism over a span of time and that the degree of change in structure produced in the nervous system by a given environmental stimulus is highly temporally related. The physician knows that all forms of learning require changes in the structure of the nervous system and, because a person both learns and forgets, it is obvious that many of the changes are reversible. Simple testing of the behavior of the system shows that the structure is very different in the baby, in the young adult, and in the old man. To no one's surprise, there is relation between the use made of the parts of the system and structure of the system. In an uncorrected strabismus, useful vision will be lost from the eye in which cortical representation is suppressed to avoid double vision. Beyond a certain age, the modification in structure caused by sensory input becomes less effective, and learning new material becomes more difficult.

We find the same variations in structure of the nervous system that we find in hearts, lungs, kidneys, skin and, in fact, in all pieces of biological systems. Some persons are color-blind, some learn tunes with difficulty, some can sort a large variety of incoming signals and distribute the information efficiently to a limited number of motor connections; others cannot effectively inhibit the spread of impulses, and many stimuli cause a widespread discharge; some extract information from the environment which is within the limits of the distribution curve of average subjects; others extract highly diverse information depending on the sensitivity of the intake apparatus, the degree of inhibition of spread, the amount of amplification, and the integration of the new information with previous information. At any point in time, the structure of the system can be tested by the behavior of the system. When the system has the first approximation of no change, repetitive and diverse testing will give similar response.

The degree of reversible change in the nervous system is easily demonstrated by repetitive stimulation of the nervous system each morning. If one massages the carotid sinus each morning in a series of patients who are standing upright, he will elicit a range of responses from no change in pulse, blood pressure, and consciousness to profound bradycardia, fall in arterial pressure, and loss of consciousness. In many patients, there is a wide variation in response from day to day. Fatigue, loss of sleep, and infection will all change the sensitivity of the system.

The fact that the integrated behavior of the patient is a reflection of the structure of the organism at one point in time allows the physician to use behavioral information for subgrouping just as he uses other data from the conventional medical history, the physical examination, and the laboratory. The chemist analyzes his material by a series of chromatographic runs in a number of solvents at varying hydrogen-ion concentrations and in both charged and uncharged fields. The physician observes the behavior of the patient as he moves through the multiple situations and experiences of life. The physician uses the data from the life chromatogram just as the chemist uses the data from the one in his laboratory. Like systems run at the same speed in all solvents, at all hydrogen-ion concentrations, and in charged and uncharged fields. Unlike systems behave differently.

The physician therefore watches his patient for any information which will define the characteristics of the system. He knows that the response of the system is limited at any one time by the structure. The structure is modifiable by normal development, by the effects of use (training, education), by many environmental influences (heat, cold, alcohol, drugs), by many disease processes (hyperadrenalism, myxedema, atherosclerosis), and by aging. These changes in structure are detected when the same stimulus produces a different response.

The appreciation that behavior has a structural basis is useful to the physician. He appreciates that habits are structurally determined and that it takes time to properly groove the nervous system. Once a habit is formed, it is modified with difficulty because it is laid down in structure. Once the cause of the difficulty in changing behavior is understood, the physician becomes less demanding of his patient. He knows that any machine looks good when it is used to perform the task for which it is best fitted. Any machine appears poorly designed when it is asked to perform outside certain limits. A fine infrared recording instrument will be only a source of trouble if one continually tries to analyze changes in the ultraviolet spectrum.

The knowledge that behavior is tightly tied to structure will prevent the physician's being surprised to learn that different members of a family interact differently with their environment. Knowing that each system has a different intake, a different route of transmission, different connections within the system, and different storage systems, he will not expect the same input into the system to be handled in the same way. He will know that a knowledge of input into the system will allow no prediction of the changes which may be produced in any particular nervous system. To determine what happens in the system, one must have some projection from the system which is capable of analysis. The response of the heart beat to a charged word, the blush which comes with embarrassment, the material written on an examination, the cold, moist palm during an interview, and the behavior of the person while driving a car yield data on the effect of the stimulus on the system.

As might be expected, some systems are so distorted that the presence of abnormalities is obvious to all. In others, the differences are more subtle. One child may learn easily to handle abstract mathematical concepts and yet learn music with difficulty. Another child will learn to read easily and well but will extract little information from social contacts with other children. One child may be a skilled musician but be color-blind.

By education and training we attempt to recognize those areas which are structured in such a way that learning is easy (so-called "natural aptitude") and those areas where learning will occur only with a large input of energy. In these second areas, we frequently need to develop cues which allow us to partially bypass the deficiencies in structure. We have to determine the amounts of energy which can be profitably invested in the areas of less competence because of the expense of special education.

We all recognize that in certain persons structure may so limit usual development that the patient will be incapacitated. Intelligence-quotient testing may show no limitation in the intellectual field, but observation demonstrates that the patient does not accumulate average information from the usual experiences of life. He clearly needs special instruction so that he can relate with his nervous sytem, the programming of which is not average to the patterns of what we call acceptable behavior. The cause of the deviations in behavior may be primary changes in the nervous system (color blindness) or the changes in the nervous system secondary to disease elsewhere (myxedema). The deviations may express themselves in socially unacceptable behavior or in a variety of somatic complaints.

The role of the physician then is to identify the structure of his patient and to determine under which circumstances he gives optimal performance. If the physician can modify the structure favorably by either medicine, surgery, or training, he will increase the capabilities of the patient. If he cannot modify the structure, he must gain acceptance by the patient of the limitation which the structure gives and have the patient live within these limitations. The practice of medicine largely sums up to 1) definition of the structure, 2) tolerance for its limitations, and 3) avoidance of situations in which this particular structure performs poorly.

It is not surprising that these same techniques which are useful in the practice of medicine are also applicable to the activities of a medical educator. Students, interns and residents come to us for training. Each is different and each gains satisfaction in different ways. Our role is not to stamp out residents from a common mold. It is rather to identify the best use of the man and to define the limits imposed by structure. *The basic patterns are well laid down by the time we meet the student.* Definition of structure, tolerance, and avoidance are dominant ways in which we plan our programs. The faculty of Duke University Medical School has certain characteristics which result primarily from selection. True enough, some modification of the reversible portions of neurogenic DNA occurs, but the overall patterns of organization, the interrelations of one part to another, and the potential of the system are already fully determined long before the person joins the faculty.

A knowledge of the tie between structure and behavior allows the biologically minded physician to devise useful social structures. He knows of the continual change in structure and appreciates the fact that each person in an organization will undergo change. He builds a social system which allows for this change. He knows that the young and old are made differently, and he requires different things from them at different times of life.

The physician who wanders among the sick and the well with an alert, curious, tolerant eye will know many things about the structure of his patients which are not learned from conventional system reviews, physical examination, and laboratory tests. He will take pleasure in observing the complexities of biology and the differences among patients. He will appreciate the limitations of extrapolation in dealing with systems which are only partially characterized. He will draw satisfactions from his ability to observe and understand the structure of the organism as demonstrated by appropriate testing, even though he cannot predict accurately the structure in advance of the testing.[4]

•

Long after the fever is gone, changes in structure may persist. It should be obvious that people don't get well at once. In a sick person, many changes take place that require some time to return to normal. It has always intrigued me that so many doctors hold on to the naive notion that once an underlying defect is controlled, the patient is well.[1]

•

It is nice to have all people equal in front of the law. This is not so in biology.

•

The biologic potentialities of man are determined by the arrangements of the purine and pyrimidine bases in the chromosomes of the cell resulting from the union of the egg and sperm. The degree to which these biologic potentials are realized is a function of the environment. A knowledge of the interplay between these two forces which determine the structure and function of mankind is of obvious importance to the physician.

The data reduction system used in the storage of information in the chromosomes is not known. It obviously exceeds that envisioned in the present or future by the IBM company. We know that the complete instructions for synthesizing all of the materials found in the body and for their orderly inter-relations are present. Each enzyme in the body appears to be controlled by one gene. Since most reactions in the body are catalyzed by a series of enzymatic reactions, the absence of one enzyme may have multiple effects. Enzymes acting further along in the process may appear to be absent because proper substrate for their activity may not appear. The products of metabolism normally changed rapidly by the missing enzyme may accumulate in the body and poison one or more enzymes not involved in the original reaction. The lack of the end products of the reaction may lead to failure of normal feedback control with overproduction of various materials.

The discovery that genes control the quantity or quality of the proteins in the body has given a more quantitative concept to the terms *dominant* and *recessive*. A protein may carry out its necessary function when it is present in only 50% of its normal concentration. Thus, the TD genotype produces the same phenotype as the TT genotype. The quantitative aspects of genotypic change is nicely shown in sickle cell anemia. Here the AS genotype produces a phenotype not greatly different from that produced by the AA genotype. When the red cells of the AS genotype are developed, it is clear that there is a smaller amount of A hemoglobin than is present in normal cells and that there is present a new hemoglobin: hemoglobin S. Nevertheless, the amount of A hemoglobin is sufficient to maintain the function of the red cells and, in general, the development of the AS body is normal. The SS genotype causes a striking change in the phenotype, which we are all familiar with as sickle cell anemia.

When we consider the amount of information which is stored in the chromosomes and the number of molecules which must be precisely arranged to give identical information, we are not surprised to discover, with the exception of identical twins, that no chromosomes contain exactly the same genes arranged in exactly the same order. This variability in genetic constitution accounts for the obvious differences we see in all persons. It accounts for the fact that we are different enough to have different names and that we can identify each other by our physical characteristics and by our behavior. These external physical and behavioral differences are the expression of the many biochemical differences which are present in each of us. These clinical differences are the expression of the genetic arrangement of the DNA in our various chromosomes.

For the physician then, modern genetics highlights the fact that every organism is an individual with its own biological potentialities. The role of the physician is to identify these individual characteristics and to modify the environment in such a way that the desirable potentials are fully developed and the undesirable potentials minimized. He knows that, from the beginning, every organism is different and that this difference will be accentuated by environmental factors.

In medicine we are confronted with an additional fact: no organism remains the same from microsecond to microsecond. We know this from the number of molecules present in the body and their complexity. It is clear that from one instant to the next we are different. Accepting the undoubted fact that we are continually changing, the practical question becomes: when does the change become different enough to modify the behavior of the biological systems which we know as Mary Jones or Tom Smith? Certain of the changes are obvious. We know that the premature baby cannot regulate his temperature, that the advent of puberty causes widespread physical and emotional changes, and that the menopause produces a variety of changes.

The continual change which occurs in the body and the difficulty of reduplicating the first approximation of the same structure is well shown in the patient who has an epileptic seizure at infrequent intervals. If he has a seizure only once a year, this means that only once yearly does the sum of his body structure and functions reach the conditions necessary for a spontaneous seizure. The same conclusion can be drawn for the patient who has a rare bout of unexplained auricular fibrillation. We now know that the structure as well as the function of a contracted muscle is different from that of a relaxed muscle.

The implication of modern genetics is that all biologic machines are structured differently and the implication of all modern physiology is that each differently structured machine is undergoing continual change.

We have already indicated that the inherent potential of the organism is genetically determined but that the final structure and function of the organism will be determined by the way that environment plays on the genetic potential. In genetic language, the phenotype is the result of the interaction of the environment on the genes.

This concept is, of course, familiar to us all. An oak tree on the rocky shores of the Pacific Coast beaten by the full force of the wind may be small and gnarled, yet its acorns will grow a stately oak in a more favorable environment.

As the years have gone by, we have realized how much the genetic possibilities can remain masked in the absence of the proper environmental stimulus. The child with galactosemia will thrive normally if milk is avoided. The middle-aged man will not develop diabetes if his weight is controlled. The primaquine-sensitive person will not develop anemia if he does not come in contact with the drug; the susceptible infant will not develop goiter if soybean milk is not used.

In clinical medicine we try to identify how the particular organism (our patient) differs from all other persons. We try to identify the factors which limit his performance. We try to find the peculiarities which make one type of living more desirable for him than others. In general, we go about this in the following way:

1. We take a family history which helps identify some of the genetic peculiarities of the patient and the effects of certain types of environmental stress on this type of genetic structure.
2. We carry out a physical examination to determine in what ways he differs from the average person.
3. We measure a number of physiologic and biochemical functions, again in an attempt to find out how he differs from others.
4. We listen to his account of the effects of stress, physical and emotional, on the ability of his body to function normally. From the history alone we may define the fact that he does well in certain situations and poorly in others. We do not have to understand the reasons for each of these peculiarities to put this information to therapeutic use. All of us can tell whether a car will start on a cold day even though we have little knowledge of the actual working of the automobile.

Our therapeutic approach is based on the following considerations:

1. Since all the machines are made differently and since each has been modified in different ways by the wear of life, they do not have equal capacities or equal uses. If we can determine the situations under which the organism functions best, we can make its performance improve. No worker in the laboratory would attempt to measure infrared rays with an instrument sensitive only to the ultraviolet. Just as each laboratory instrument has its limitations, so does each organism.
2. Knowing that the machine has limitations in areas of physical performance, intellectual work, and in emotional adjustments to complex situations, and that these limitations are permanent and are characteristic of the person, we are willing to accept the

limitations and not expect of the patient performances which are clearly impossible for him. Every wife discovers that her husband behaves in certain ways which seem irrational to her but which are part of him and are not susceptible to change. The husband learns the same thing about his wife.

Men are not free to do everything. The bonds of heredity and the grooves worked by environment allow little play, and the behavior of man is remarkably repetitious. Knowledge that these limitations are not self-imposed but are a reflection of the overall biological processes present allow us to be patient with persons who present us with problems which are difficult to solve, and this reflection helps us to recognize that care of particular patients may be easy or difficult but that patients cannot be divided into good patients and bad patients.

3. Having identified the areas where the patient breaks down under stress, we can do the following:
   a. Strengthen the part if possible by improving mechanical parts or by adding material which is lacking.
   b. Avoid the stress. What is stress for the particular patient has to be learned by observation.
   c. If we elect not to avoid the stress and protect a weak area, then pay the bill cheerfully. [1961]

•

Under some circumstances, some machines will freeze and under other circumstances, some machines will boil over. What we haven't yet learned to cope with is the fact that, as the level of competence necessary to achieve independence is raised, more machines are going to freeze or boil over.[1]

•

As he watches in man the changes with age, the physician becomes aware that flexibility is continually dropping out of the system. The man at 50 is a markedly different man from the man at 30.[5]

•

Good Will Toward Men: Christmas is coming and our thoughts turn toward ways of making this a better world. None of us knows how to bring about "peace on earth" but each of us can contribute to the ideal of "good will toward men". The family doctor, by the breadth of his experience and by his dealing with life in all its phases and with the death which comes to each of us, has the best opportunity to develop the deep understanding of human behavior and tolerance of biologic phenomena which truly allow him to manifest "good will toward men".

The understanding doctor does not divide his patients into "good" or "bad" patients. He knows that each man has a structure that is peculiar to

him and that the structure of any person at any one point in time is the
result of the interactions of genetic and environmental factors. He can
identify similarities and differences between one man and another by
observing the reactions of each to a wide variety of common stimuli.
Identical structures give identical responses to a common stimulus and
non-identical ones give different responses. The doctor knows that the
behavior of any biologic organism at any one point in time reflects the
structure of the organism. Behavior does not occur by magic or in a
vacuum. It is the expression of the integrated structure of the organism.

A knowledge of the obligatory tie between structure and behavior is
important to the doctor who has to deal with human behavior all day long.
The structure and therefore the behavior of the body change rapidly in
embryo and slowly in old age. The changes in structure may be reversible
or irreversible. The retina of the dark-adapted eye has a different structure
from the light-adapted eye. The sleeping man differs from the waking man.
The heart of a person taking digitalis is different from the heart before the
administration of digitalis. These differences in structure are not definable
by the usual method of tissue examination, but chemical analysis will
define differences. It is easier, of course, to determine that differences exist
by observing the reactions of the retina in the two states to light, by testing
the reflexes of the awake and sleeping man, and by observing the reactions
of the predigitalized and the digitalized heart to different concentrations of
potassium. There are many non-reversible differences in structure. The
changes in nuclear DNA in the mongoloid, the destroyed kidney of glomerulonephritis, the number of neurons in the central nervous system, the
length of the adult femur are not reversible.

The doctor discovers that habits are bedded in the structure of the
nervous system. They cannot be formed with repetition and they cannot be
eliminated rapidly without destroying a portion of the nervous system. The
doctor does not lightly ask his patient to change a lifelong pattern of living.
He knows that changes in the structure of the nervous system are increasingly difficult to initiate in later years and that the old patterns cannot
be eliminated without a considerable investment of energy. He is careful to
select out the few really important things that he wants done and to devote
all of his skill to seeing that enough energy is put into the system to
establish such new patterns.

The constant awareness of the obligatory tie between structure and
behavior keeps the doctor alert to the importance of determining the best
fit between the patient and his environment. Every instrument (and here
we include man as an instrument) operates within definable limits, and any

instrument used within these limits gives its best performance. A photocell designed to react in the infrared will not perform well with ultraviolet light; a tone-deaf man makes a poor musician. Every person is a different instrument and operates best when used within his own particular limits. The extent that one person differs from another must be defined by observing the similarities and differences in behavior to a wide variety of situations. One is not dependent on the formal medical history, the physical examination and the usual laboratory studies to define similarities and differences. A chemist determines the similarities and differences between two peptides by observing the speed of movement of each peptide in a variety of solvents in both charged and uncharged fields. The environment is the solvent in which man runs to write a lifelong chromatogram. The doctor defines the similarities and differences between two persons by observing their reactions to a common environment over a number of years.

The appreciation of the link between structure and behavior accounts for the doctor's tolerance. He does not expect all things from all men. Structure is only in part reversible by environment and training. The doctor can accept realistically and without malice the necessary compromises that his patients force him to make in therapy because the structure of the patients makes ideal behavior impossible. The doctor cannot, at present, reverse the changes of chronic myocardial fibrosis. He cannot reverse the structural basis responsible for color blindness or for the inability to learn how others feel during usual social contacts.

There are people who make significant contributions to society and others who are destructive to society. The fortunate folk who perform well tend to take personal credit for their fine performance and to look with some disdain on those who perform less well. In reality, the good performers are due no personal credit. Their DNA and favorable environmental forces have molded a machine which functions well to meet the needs of the current society. Make the necessary changes in their nervous and endocrine systems and they will quickly become useless to society, and no amount of "will power" will counteract the structural change. The person disdained by society is also a physical machine whose structure has been determined by the interaction of his DNA and his environment. He will remain useless unless some change in structure occurs. He is not a bad man. He merely represents a poorly built machine.

If one wishes to change the behavior of man, one must change the anatomy of his nervous system. Purposeful modification of human DNA will not occur for many years. Favorable changes in the next generation must come from modifications of structure produced by manipulation of environment. Better nutrition of parents, prevention of infections and bio-chemical changes unfavorable to the fetus, better nutrition and living conditions for infants and children, improved techniques for training and educating the young so that patterns useful for both intellectual and social purposes will be formed in the central nervous system offer us our best chance to mold the anatomy of the nervous system of our future generations.

Will many of our yet-to-be-born children lack the optimal chance for favorable development? Will lack of proper nutrition and health and lack of properly timed stimuli to mold the nervous system hamper the growth of children? We know that unfortunately the answer is "yes!". All of us would like to change that answer. The question is how. Let the spirit of Christmas inspire in each of us his own best answer.[6]

•

This concept of the relationship between behavior and structure is of particular importance to doctors dealing with patients with chronic illness. By definition, these persons have difficulties great enough to separate them from persons we call well. They have either lost part of their ability to adjust to external environment and to maintain a constant environment, or they have organs sufficiently sensitive to small changes so that the patient is repetitively made aware of minute changes in internal or external environ-ment. The illness itself alters their position in the family, in the community and in their occupation. Any feelings which are caused by these changed relationships cause changes in their bodies. At present, the magnitude of these changes is better shown by the behavior of the patient than by biochemical tests or x-rays. The reversibility of many of these changes in structure can be established by the reversibility of the behavior under treatment by a trained health team.

. . . During this period of time the doctor also learns of the tremendous alterations in structure which are produced by the sensory stimuli, by emotional content of thought and by changes in physical environment. When he sees a normal person, adjusting rapidly to maintain a normal external environment, he may not appreciate the extent of the changes. The body effectively buffers the effects of the stimulus so that the stimulus appears to the observer to be a weak one. In reality, the stimulus may be a potent one and may appear inert only because of the effective counter-forces mobilized by the body. As disease or time-dependent processes change the body, or as environmental changes favorable to activating potential genetic weakness occur, one becomes more aware of the force of many previously unappreciated stimuli. Destroy the sympathetic nervous system and the patient loses consciousness on standing. Destroy the lung by emphysema and a small dose of nembutal may produce fatal respiratory failure. Alter the heart by amyloid and the changes in the body brought about by apprehension of a chest tap may produce fatal pulmonary edema. The bronchial mucosa of an asthmatic person may detect changes in structure initiated by certain interpersonal contacts or social situations as delicately as the string galvanometer picks up the electrical current initiating the heart beat.[5]

* * * *

When you put the CNS into the cycle, you don't have to have a 1:1 relation between the stimulus and the subjective response.

•

The dying in cardiovascular disease is determined by the heart. What one does when he has cardiovascular disease is determined by the brain.

•

You have to know the culture of the system as well as the science of the system in order for things to work at all.

•

I have always thought that hysteria was one of the normal central nervous system patterns like sleep, rather than an illness. It is more likely to be apparent in sick people, just as anoxia is in sickle cell disease.[1]

•

Learning from clinical experience is not simple. Patients differ in their biological potentialities. Many factors of importance in clinical medicine become obvious only when they are tested in a particular portion of the population under appropriate circumstances. The biological system changes and there are dangers in using the same patient as his own control. When the biology of the patient is sufficiently altered, past experiences may be misleading rather than helpful.

The nervous system is an amplifying system. One cannot gauge the intensity of the sensory stimuli entering the system by the degree of disturbance that the stimuli cause.

The most common factor that drives a patient to a doctor is anxiety. An accurate evaluation of the problem is not possible unless the effect of this force is properly evaluated.

Doctors learn at two levels: 1) the scientific, when the variables can be properly controlled, and 2) experiential, frequently without understanding, when the variables are uncontrolled.

•

People do not have freedom at any one time to determine exactly how they feel about something. At any one time, the body has limitations with regard to its feeling states and behavior. The limitations are two: 1) the point of maximum limit, and 2) certain reversible pieces. People don't appreciate the biological basis of behavior.

•

Denial has some value. Don't get mad at it, just understand that it occurs.

•

It has long been recognized that patients with spontaneous or exercise-produced hyperventilation have irritable nervous systems. The fact that the respiratory center does not slow down respiration when enough CO_2 has been lost to produce alkalosis is a sign of incoordination in the regulation of respiration. The patient may be taught to recognize the symptoms of hyperventilation and he may prevent them by breathing into a closed container, as a paper bag, but he will not recover normal smooth control of respiration unless the nervous system functions more normally. He can learn to understand his symptoms and tolerate them and be interested in the situations producing them, but this will not prevent uneven respiratory regulation in times of stress.

The patient with this kind of symptomatology is usually telling the physician two things: 1) his sensory nervous system is unusually sensitive to changes in environment so that changes commonly ignored are now noticed, and 2) homeostatic regulation is poor so that swings in the internal environment are greater than normal. Both are responsible for a rather diffuse symptomatology. Examination of the patient shows that he has many evidences of poor homeostatic control. He has cold hands and feet, he sweats profusely in certain areas, goose flesh appears and disappears, and the blood pressure rises too high at times and frequently falls more than expected under the stress of standing. History confirms irregular function of the gastrointestinal tract and the bladder, and the difficulty in sexual activities. The laboratory shows both high and low concentrations of blood sugar, the cholesterol varies, and the electrocardiogram is unstable.

The physician is likely to attribute the symptoms to the area of his own greatest interest. If he is studying the phenomenon of hyperventilation, this will be the diagnosis. If he is interested in blood sugar regulation, he will believe that he has an instance of functional hypoglycemia. If he is interested in postural reactions, he will attribute considerable importance to the fall in pressure on standing. If he is a gastroenterologist, he will be struck by many similarities between his patient and the "dumping syndrome." If he is a cardiologist, he will be intrigued by the changing electrocardiographic pattern. Because of the dyspnea and the marked changes in pulse rate, he will summarize his impressions by the diagnosis of "effort syndrome."

In time, the physician is impressed with how little the basic complaint is helped by attention to one aspect of this diffuse disturbance, and he realizes that the patient is describing his overall problem in sensory pickup and regulation of body function, and not a specific disturbance in a single function. He then needs to know what do doctors know about this type of illness and what is its course.

Some persons are born with a sensitive nervous system in which impulses "sprangle" (a fine Carolina term), and in which most sensory impulses cause widespread motor discharges. These patients may always be conscious of their body and the changes in their internal environment. Once they learn about their makeup, they should approach the doctor with the question: "Are these sensations disease or is this I?" Both patient and doctor have to recognize the biologic organization of these particular patients and not be irritated because it differs from others.

The fact that patients are able, by their wide testing of themselves in the stresses of living, to find out that their bodies have changed when all of the physician's laboratory findings show no change is not surprising. The patient is reporting the results of a series of biologic assays, and we know from experience that many biologic assays have a sensitivity far beyond that of our present chemical methods. In addition to this difficulty, we do not know all of the active ingredients of any biologic system. Therefore, it is not surprising that the patient describes to us symptoms that we do not understand.

Our knowledge of the symptomatology produced by discrete lesions in the nervous system is still in its infancy. As one watches the changes which occur in an aging population, it is clear that many of their reactions are determined by central nervous system disease. Many of the mechanisms of homeostasis which are reversibly disturbed in the person without destructive disease in the nervous system are permanently crippled in patients with destructive changes in the nervous system. In the early stage of destructive illness, symptomatology may be diffuse and hyperventilation may be present. Only a long followup will determine the kind of illness we are dealing with.[7]

* * * *

People have anxiety attacks which they interpret as heart attacks. If the doctor knows the patient has no heart trouble, he calls them anxiety attacks. How rarely in the patient with known heart disease does the differential diagnosis include anxiety attacks!

* * * *

Many patients go from doctor to doctor thinking that they are sick, and are never told that they are really well in a way they can understand. If a hundred people listen to a Beethoven symphony, some will be in ecstasy and some will be bored. These are not good and bad people, but people with different central nervous systems. Some people interpret almost all signals from their central nervous systems as signs of sickness. They are not sick, but just have different receivers.

•

It is not enough to know that poverty, insecurity and perhaps poor vocational and domestic relations are now keeping the patient unhappily depressed, for all too often it is apparent that present socio-economic factors are not crucial determinants in the contemporary scene. To explain the phenomena, it is necessary to remember that past experiences of each individual from earlier days are not altogether forgotten but are foundations on which rest his current system of meeting daily problems. Under pressure, some of the defensive attitudes useful in infancy and childhood, but inappropriate in adult life, have a way of returning to the scene of action; one of the oldest—the state of readiness for fight or flight—may be the precipitating cause of illness such as peptic ulcer or hypertension when called upon too frequently.

* * * *

I've never understood why patients in hospitals are given sedatives for anxiety. This is the easiest way to cloud the sensorium and the problem.[1]

•

The more well you are, the more drugs you can take without getting sick. That's why doctors don't get into more trouble than they do with therapy.[1]

•

When you have a doctor, a patient, and a drug, there is much room for misunderstanding.[1]

* * * *

I imagine that if you could assemble 100 fat people who had dieted successfully and 100 fat people who had not, the 100 people who had not lost weight would be healthier. People who voluntarily lose weight frequently do it only after being frightened by a severe illness.[1]

•

Fat people are fat because they are more comfortable that way. The day is easier being obese than suffering from the discomforts of not eating.[1]

•

A man who loses weight from a well-planned diet is likely to have trouble with his friends. They notice that he is becoming thinner and immediately assume that he is ill.

* * * *

All symptomatology results from stimulation of the nervous system. The nervous system consists of a series of sensory pickups, a system of amplification or inhibition, and a system for motor discharges. The degree to which a given stimulus spreads through the nervous system and the degree to which it is amplified will determine the motor discharge. One cannot, therefore, measure the sensory input by the intensity of the motor discharge. This results in the situation familiar to all physicians but a source of surprise to many patients: you can't tell how ill you are by how bad you feel.

All body functions are regulated by oscillating systems. The body has no mechanism for regulating along a straight line. When the oscillating swings regulating homeostasis are wide, afferent stimuli entering the nervous system are increased and the patient becomes aware of his body and complains of various symptoms. The number of afferent impulses that are fed into the nervous system affect in turn the sensitivity of the system.

The extent of the oscillations and the sensitivity of the nervous system determine the degree of complaining. These variables are in part genetic in origin, but they are influenced by many other factors, in both health and disease.

•

All of the problems of getting through the day become magnified when you are ill.

•

A patient comes to a doctor with a complaint. The first problem the doctor must solve is complex: is his patient ill or well? The patient's complaint may arise because 1) a well body is equipped with a sensitive nervous system which detects changes induced in everyone by environment which are not detected by less sensitive systems; or 2) a well body is being used in a way which would make most bodies complain; or 3) the patient's nondiseased but nevertheless highly individualized body is being used in a way that would not make *most* well bodies complain but does make his well, though somewhat different, body complain; or 4) illness is raising its ugly head.

. . . The patient going to the doctor with complaints commonly assumes that he is ill. If the doctor prescribes medication or other therapy without carefully distinguishing—to the patient as well as himself—when he is caring for the patient as a healthy person with complaints and when he is treating illness, the patient's assumption of illness is reinforced. The reality of the complaining is not the point at issue. The question is: is illness the cause of the complaining? The fact that this question is not easy to answer simply means doctoring is difficult.[8]

•

I don't know any pain that nervousness doesn't make worse, do you?

•

Our system is always biased because we're getting the complaining part of the population.

•

For 20 years, in hypertension the symptoms are not related to the hypertension, and I have to realize this or the medicine becomes very screwy.

•

If you are going to treat or subject a patient to a long period of therapy, it's important to know whether he is actually sick or not. It becomes obvious if a person works long hours on his feet that his feet will become tired and ache at the end of the day. This doesn't mean that his legs are bad.

•

It is very easy in clinical medicine to double-weight evidence. Over 20 years, every time the patient came in, the diagnosis of rheumatic fever became more definite.

•

[*To a scared young female patient on rounds*]: Let me tell you one nice thing about being young. When you get sick, you're going to get well. We don't know what you've got but we know you're going to get better.

* * * *

Sick systems are not like healthy systems. People die in pieces.[1]

•

I have a bird in the house; he looks well. I walk into the house, he is frightened, hits the glass and dies. There are many ways in which the nervous system kills you.

•

The nearer you get to being dead, the less anything works.

•

People cannot get well in one of two ways: either they continue in the same state or they die.

•

People don't die in hospitals from lack of food or water but they do from aspiration.[1]

•

There are many different patterns of dying. In a hospital it is a social affair. People are continually doing what good people are expected to do in this setting.

•

Death solves problems for some. For some, death takes two weeks; for others 30 years. All are uncomfortable about it—the three of us: the patient, the spouse and the doctor.

•

The thing you try to do in dying is leave the fewest scars behind. The dying patient solves his problem: he dies. It's the living that are left behind that you must pay attention to.

•

By reading the obituary pages . . . we discover that professors of preventive medicine and leaders of the American Heart Association die at the same age as their unscientific business associates. [1967]

•

Living was, in years past, looked upon as a natural phenomenon largely under the control of Providence and little influenced by the actions of man. Dying, except from violence or poisoning, was looked upon also as an inevitable phenomenon, with the time of the dying beyond the control of man. These attitudes are now obsolete. Today man has much more control over the time of dying. This change, produced by medical science, is causing us to examine more closely the ethical and legal framework of living and dying.

With us always has been the question of when the life of the individual begins and when society begins to protect this life because it has gained the dignity of a human being. Eggs and sperm die separately without any pangs of conscience. The "pill", as commonly used, prevents ovulation and does not cause the death of the fertilized egg. When the egg and sperm unite, a process is initiated which will produce a highly individualized unique person. The "pill" can be used in large doses to prevent implantation of the fertilized egg. What are the ethical and legal complications of this use of the "pill"?

The doctor has always accepted the responsibility that the survival of frank monsters is not in the best interest of society, and no unusual means are employed to keep them alive. Many mentally defective children have correctable associated defects. Correction of these defects, particularly when they involve the cardiovascular system, may prolong life for many years without modifying mental capacity. What frames of reference should the doctor use in determining in which of these children corrective surgery should be done?

Death was once an agreed-upon endpoint. This has ceased to be true. Every day, persons in whom the heart and respiration have stopped are restored to life and return to normal activity. On the other hand, we have patients who are still alive because the heart and respiration continue though the brain has ceased to function. What is the current legal definition of death?

The medical profession is trained to save life. If a condemned criminal is hurt before the time for his execution, a team of doctors and nurses will work all night to keep him alive and restore him to health. The doctor's instinct is to prolong life. He has seen many people recover from desperate situations. He has seen many people die after prolonged efforts. He has seen great hardships result from keeping alive persons who can never again contribute to family life or to society. How do the doctor and the patient's family determine when the doctor should become passive?

Depressed patients may commit suicide. If this can be prevented, most patients will recover. All doctors agree that prevention of suicide of a depressed patient is a responsibility of the medical profession. What legal and ethical considerations should guide the physician when a non-depressed patient attempts to take his own life because he faces dishonor or incurable illness?

Patients under Medicare are supported in our hospital only as long as they can be shown to continue to profit by the care. Most ill patients will live longer if they remain in the hospital than if they are sent to a nursing home. How does the doctor determine at what point Medicare benefits stop? In past years these matters were usually determined administratively by the county commissioners. It was their responsibility to discontinue funds for hospitalization and they were not usually overly concerned that, without hospitalization, death would occur sooner. Now these decisions are being placed more and more often with the doctor. What legal and ethical considerations guide the hospital utilization committee in such decisions?

To what degree does the patient or the family control medical treatment and when does society make the decision which may disregard the wishes of the individual? Most will agree that adults who are rational can decide their own fate. The matter becomes more difficult when minors are involved. Should a child in danger of dying from hemorrhage receive a transfusion if it is against the wishes of the family? Who should make the decision and on what grounds?

The successful development of intensive care units for patients with myocardial infarction and the successful treatment of previously fatal kidney failure raise the most acute problems about the role of society in the problems of living and dying.

Many patients are alive and active today because of the prompt use of external cardiac massage, electrical defibrillation and mouth-to-mouth breathing. There is suggestive evidence that coronary care units not only can restore the dead to life but, by careful monitoring and proper use of drugs, can prevent the change in cardiac rhythm that will cause death. These units are expensive. They create enormous demands for trained manpower. How much of the resources of the country should be devoted to the care of the population beyond the age of 40 who clearly have a limited life expectancy when compared to the neglected, preschool child of three?

The time of dying of patients with kidney failure is now largely an administrative matter. Renal dialysis and transplantation would allow additional years of life for many of our patients. Each such life prolonged for a year or more represents a large investment of money and manpower..The program raises many ethical considerations. Does every man so love his brother that he will give him one kidney? Kidneys of people who die can be used for transplantation if they are promptly harvested after death.

This takes agreement and planning during the life of the donor. What protection does the donor have that his own life will not be shortened to benefit the recipient? Should the organs of a dead man belong to the family or to society?[9]

•

There are no great thoughts beyond death, as far as I know. If there are, no one has ever presented them.

* * * *

Optimal health services are that degree of care which allows the individual to discharge his role in society with the minimal restrictions from preventable and curable illness and with the best compromises that can be made with nonpreventable and noncurable illnesses. What is optimal health care for one is not optimal health care for another.

We can agree reasonably well on what is optimal care for infants, children and pregnant women. It is clear that more medical care alone will not solve the problems of poverty, poor housing, slothfulness, illiteracy, drunkenness and lack of a family structure. Nevertheless we can agree on standards of optimal care for the infants, the children and the mothers, and we can document whether or not this care was given.

In the adult group we have more difficulty both in defining medical care and in determining what medical and nonmedical factors prevent the individual from receiving optimal medical care. Any obese person, smoking cigarettes and driving his car away from a cocktail party is clearly receiving less than optimal health care. He may well have been offered good services but he has clearly declined them.

Finally, there are certain situations in which optimal medical care requires the use of particular procedures because of the occupation of the patient.

Sudden death or hemiplegia in an airplane pilot may kill a hundred persons. Optimal health care of pilots cannot, in good judgment, be equated with optimal health care for school teachers, for instance.

The records of the public services of our teaching hospitals are not very useful in establishing a baseline for optimal health care overall. The teaching hospitals are concerned primarily with the conversion of raw manpower into skilled manpower for use in the health professions. The records that are kept, the diagnostic procedures that are ordered, and the treatments administered are designed primarily to meet the needs of manpower production. The impact of such health services on the individual patient who is functioning poorly in our society is not great because cultural, economic, social, and educational deficiencies prevent the operation at home of the schedules carefully worked out in the hospital.[10]

•

Ten percent of the population use 90% of the medical facilities. This is the reason why medical insurance works.[1]

•

Today, with periodic pre-employment and insurance examinations, the scope of the physician has been enlarged. He must be accomplished in the study of presumedly well people in addition to those who are ill. With the latter group, the history is of great value; with those who are well, objective methods of study are all important, for patients tend to emphasize different facts, depending on whether they seek employment, pensions, disability, or insurance. It is obvious that the same symptoms will rarely be described in the same way by the soldier desiring release from military duty, by the prospective employee seeking certification of his fitness for work or by the patient who is alarmed because of fear of a serious illness. The approach to the patient therefore must be varied to correspond to the conditions which bring physician and patient together.[1]

REFERENCES

1. Schoonmaker F, Metz E. Just Say For Me. World Press Inc., Denver, 1968.
2. Stead EA. Medical Times 95: 802, 1967.
3. Stead EA. Arch. Int. Med. 127: 703, 1971.
4. Stead EA. Billings Lecture. J. A. M. A. 195: 157, 1966.
5. Stead EA. Ann. Int. Med. 110: 409, 1962.
6. Stead EA. Medical Times 94: 1537, 1966.
7. Stead EA. Disease-a-Month, February 1960, pp. 5-31.
8. Stead EA. Medical Times 96: 753, 1968.
9. Stead EA. Medical Times 95: 1173, 1967.
10. Stead EA. Medical Times 95: 356, 1967.

An Era of Medical Service Has Ended

ANTICIPATION OF NEED FOR CHANGE;
PROPOSALS OF LOGICAL ALTERNATIVES

The old system in the past has been saved by making the doctor more efficient. Antibiotics were equal to a graduating class of doctors each year. The giving up of home practice resulted in a great increase in efficiency. There are no further gains to be made to allow the present supply of doctors to give the services demanded of them by persons between 55 and 80 who have not died.

It is time that the medical profession accepted the fact that *an era of medical service has ended.* Efforts to shore up the old system are doomed to failure. The solo general practitioner is gone. Group practice with specialization will be the model for the future. Each doctor must be responsible for more patients. To do this, he must have a new corps of assistants, which we have elected to call physician's assistants. These will be men recruited by doctors, trained by doctors and paid by doctors. They will be responsible for all patient care below the level of the doctor. A group in practice will use the same group of physician's assistants in the clinic, in the home and in the hospital. [1966]

•

[*To a physician who wrote concerning a shortage of medical manpower*]: The problem lies in the fact that no one takes the responsibility for all personal health services in a given area. Each doctor is responsible for his own patients. Under this philosophy, there is no incentive to extend one's efforts to care for other patients because the doctor is well paid for caring for his current patients. If the members of a county medical society would agree to supply personal health services to all the patients in the county, they would have to devise ways to meet this responsibility. My suggestion would be to award a prize to the first county medical society that devised and implemented a plan to give personal health services to all the people in its county.

•

I am not convinced that all medical practice is best done by groups. In my experience, group practice is a good arrangement for handling complex medical problems and for continuing the education of doctors. The more time the doctor has for thinking, the more expensive the medical care. There are many problems of health maintenance and primary care which can be handled effectively by patterned responses which do not require rethinking of each problem. A well-integrated solo practitioner with a good office staff can handle a large volume of problems more efficiently and more cheaply than any of the clinics I have seen.

The problem of solo practice is the lack of support for vacations, sickness and education. The appearance of the physician's assistant on the scene has put much more flexibility into the solo practitioner's day. The development of consortiums of solo practitioners and the doctors in medical centers to which they refer patients is worth careful exploration. If adequate support systems could be devised, the advantages of solo or duo practice would not be lost.

I am also less impressed with the benefits of putting all doctors on a salary and reducing the fee-for-service aspect of medicine. Some patients need more medical attention than the doctor believes they need. He gives this service willingly for a fee. He gives it grudgingly if he is on a salary. The patient isn't always wrong.

. . . Dr. Wilburt Davison commented many years ago on the distribution of senior faculty giving care to patients in the Duke Medical Center after 5:00 P.M. on week days and on Saturday afternoons and Sunday. He found that the salaried doctors were not in the patient care areas but the fee-for-service doctors were. A recent check by me shows that Dr. Davison was a good observer. The distribution in the patient care areas of the Duke Medical Center of doctors on salary and those on fee-for-service on Saturday afternoons is similar to that observed 25 years ago.[1]

•

As you know, I would have preferred the development of a health care delivery system that did not require the large expansion of medical schools. Now that this expansion has occurred, I believe that we will have so many doctors that they will never allow the development of a rational system.

•

Appreciation that the clinical material commonly learned in medical school can be effectively taught to motivated high school graduates who derive satisfaction from the delivery of personal health services and who have a reasonably rapid rate of learning opens up the health field to rural and minority groups. No progress can be expected in this area when it takes

11 years from the first day of college until the first day of practice. One of two things happens at present. Commonly, the person from the rural area or minority group just never tries to enter the system. The culture in which he has developed does not equip him to plan for an 11-year period between starting a program and reaping the rewards of his efforts. If by chance he does enter the race, he spends 11 years working with people who are alien to his culture. In order to survive, he becomes more and more like his class-mates. By the time he enters practice, he has no desire to return to the culture of his origin. We have seen this same phenomenon happen many times when students from Asia, Africa, and South America spend their college, medical school, and graduate years in the United States. They have excellent preparation for living in middleclass America, but do not thrive when they return home.[1]

•

Experience has shown me that medical students are willing to make a much greater commitment to the hard sciences and mathematics than are other health professionals. The attempt to mix medical students, nurses and physician's assistants in course work is generally unsuccessful and does not result in the development of teams which work together effectively. After all, doctors have dated nurses, courted nurses and married nurses with no effect on the professional behavior of doctors and nurses. One can more successfully mix these groups at the patient interface. The medical student will not learn introductory medicine, the methods of physical examination, electrocardiography, care of fractures, clinical pharmacology, and care of the patient with hypertension any faster than other persons with much less preparation in science. Mixing is intuitively tried early and if this fails it is never attempted again. Once more, we learn that observations are more useful than intuition. Team concepts are best learned at the doctor-patient interface, and here a team approach to patient care can be easily developed.

* * * *

Over many years, the health field paid very low wages. Sick people were less productive than well people, and the ill rapidly became indigent. The amount of training required below the level of the doctor was not great, and the positions could be filled by women who were attracted to nursing and would work for a low wage, and by untrained personnel who could not find employment elsewhere. Hospitals were largely eleemosynary institutions and were exempt from minimum wage and hour regulations. The fact that the health profession lived off the sick and could use unskilled labor established a pattern of financing that will plague the health professions for years. Society is now taking the position that persons giving health care be paid a wage above the poverty level. Society is unhappy with health care given by the untrained, but it has yet to adjust itself to the fact that a new pattern of health care designed to prevent as well as to treat illness will have a much higher cost.

The belief at Duke is that persons should be selected for training as physician's assistants who have already demonstrated an aptitude and liking for work with sick people. Many bright young men with high-school or junior college training are in the medical corps of the Navy, Army, and Air Force, and have the opportunity to determine their aptitude for the health area. Ambitious high-school graduates can work in a hospital and demonstrate their motivation and aptitude. It is not believed that a college degree is necessary to develop a highly trained and useful assistant. There is no wish to increase the cost of production of the assistant by too long a commitment to general education.

It will take two years to train effective assistants. In the first year they will acquire a working knowledge of anatomy, physiology, pharmacology, microbiology and electronics. There must be some experience with the trauma, wound healing, suturing and handling of living tissue. In the second year the assistant will learn to take a history and perform a good physical examination. He will work in the recovery room, the emergency clinic, the coronary care unit, the renal dialysis unit and the respiratory care unit. In the last part of his second year he can work in a private clinic, in a doctor's office or in the admitting service of a busy hospital. If he wishes to restrict his activity to one clinical area, his last few months may be spent in cardiology, allergy, pulmonary disease, renology, endocrinology or the emergency clinic.

The final duties of the assistant must be determined by the doctor to whom he is responsible. At the time of his graduation, the medical center will record on his certificate the skills that have been developed, and will certify that he is competent to use these skills under the direction of a physician. If the physician wants him to have additional skills, he can return him to the medical center for additional training and appropriate updating of his certificate. It is to be hoped that the physician's assistants would not themselves be licensed, but that the schools producing them would be licensed. The responsibility for not using his assistant beyond his degree of training would remain the responsibility of the doctor.[2]

•

Persons with a high-school education, a reasonable rate of learning, and a tolerance of the unavoidably irrational demands often made by sick people can learn to do well those things which the doctor does each day. Under the wing of the doctor, such a physician's assistant can collect clinical data, including the history and physical examination, organize the material in a way which allows its use in diagnosis, and carry out any required therapeutic procedure which the doctor commonly uses. He can, of course, master any technical procedure which the doctor uses frequently. In fact, as a part of the doctor's team, he performs so well that the patient cannot tell who is the assistant.[1]

•

The medical profession has never had assistance in the care of patients from a group of career-dedicated men selected, trained and paid by doctors. Selling assistants to doctors had many of the aspects of selling bathtubs in a country which had never had plumbing. What do you do with bathtubs? Similarly, what do you do with assistants?[3]

•

The reader will grasp the fact that the authors believe there is a great difference between the best-trained assistant and the best-trained doctor. We will also admit that the education of the doctor does not always achieve our theoretical ideal. It is probable that some schools and medical centers are training assistants and calling them doctors.[1]

•

The discovery by the doctor that his assistant can do on any one day the majority of things that he himself does raises some interesting questions about medical education. Why does it take so long to educate the doctor and so little time to educate the assistant?

The doctor's education consists of four parts: 1) preparation to function as a citizen, 2) language preparation so that he can obtain content as needed from books written in part in symbolic languages, 3) development of problem-solving abilities, and 4) application of known knowledge to medical practice.

The society wishes its doctors to have a reasonable knowledge of people, history, social sciences, literature, and art because the doctor must relate the mysteries of the human body to the rest of the society. Doctors care for the leaders of our society in times of trouble and, because of the nature of the doctor-patient relationship, doctors can influence the course of the society out of proportion to their actual numbers.

The natural and, hopefully, the social sciences are taught to our doctors because a knowledge of the symbolic languages developed by these disciplines makes a wide variety of content available over the doctor's lifetime. The specific content taught is not important; the ability to read books written in the language of the particular science is important.

The preclinical portion of the doctor's experience serves a third purpose—namely, to increase problem-solving abilities. Again, the content used to modify the nervous system by having it engage in problem-solving is not important. Practice in problem-solving will modify the nervous system in a favorable way so that problems, regardless of their nature, can be approached more effectively.

The application of known knowledge to the care of people is taught by the apprentice method. This method is very effective for teaching the medicine of today. If one paces the learning correctly and teaches what is not known, one can intersperse apprentice learning with problem solving, use of symbolic language, and acquisition of new content related to the medicine of tomorrow.

The overall purpose of the long educational program for the doctor is to prepare him for a lifetime of good citizenship and a lifetime of learning. The intent is to create a thinking doctor who is completely protected against obsolescence regardless of the changes in the social and technological scene.

One can make a first approximation of the success of the educational program by watching the doctor at his daily work. If he has time in the day to be thoughtful, if he can gain new content by the use of his training in symbolic language, if he is continually preparing for the medicine of tomorrow, the educational system is justified. If he is harried, tired, handling patients in a routine, non-thinking way, the educational system has failed.

I am confident that the PA can put time back into the day of the practicing physician, provided the doctor is able to organize his own day and is capable of being a good supervisor. We do not select medical students for this talent, and our clinical support system may founder on this hidden reef.

The time has come for medical schools to broaden the intake of students to include those who have done well in the areas of economics, business administration, sociology, information sciences, and bioengineering and those who wish to continue their development in these areas while they are becoming doctors. The present high and inflexible bioscience hurdles keep out of medical schools many students with special aptitudes in other areas who are unwilling to spend two years memorizing a large number of facts in bioscience in order to pass the required medical school examinations. Those who are willing to undertake the memory work usually turn out not to have been particularly interested in the areas of their undergraduate work and do not continue to develop and use those areas. For example, the engineering graduate who comes into medicine has usually rejected engineering before he enrolls in medical school. Medicine needs an input from engineering students who maintain an interest in engineering while they are becoming doctors.

In the near future some medical school is going to convert its medical center into a true university laboratory. Doctors, medical students, interns, and residents will live with the information scientist, the economist, the professor of business administration, the sociologist, and the bioengineer. They will learn the culture of sick and well persons, the ways of doctors, and the culture of medicine. The doctors in turn will know these new colleagues and will be willing to use their talents in the education of doctors. We will continue to produce our current bioscience-based product but also we will produce equally good practicing doctors with a wide diversity of interests and skills. The paths for learning the disciplines underlying the health field and the delivery of health care will be varied. At the research level, the student's experiences will reflect his interest, and the doctor with a bioscience base will engage in quite different areas of research than the doctor with the information-science base. The non-bioscience-based doctor will be as effective in patient care as his bioscience-based colleague.[4]

* * * *

I would like to say a word about the names in the health profession. They do get us in trouble. People look on a physician with an M.D. as a kind of a uniform product, when actually you know M.D.s are no longer interchangeable. They have a very wide spectrum of activities, and therefore determining how many doctors there are in relation to population gives you no information at all about the numbers of people who are available for any particular kind of things which physicians do.

Now we are even in worse trouble in regard to nurses. You know if you use the word "nurse" it gives a fairly uniform picture to the physician and to many of the consumers of health care. But, interestingly enough, this picture is quite different from the picture the word "nurse" means to the nursing educator. We would have to say, at least in our part of the world, nursing education is becoming a general form of education. And I would have to say that we have a very attractive student body. They are fun to talk to and to work with. They generally marry well and they live well. But they are no longer a very active force in the health field. And, because of the amount of time which is devoted to general education in the course of the relatively short half-life of active work in the field, we do not any longer look upon the nurse as a primary person allied with the physician who is going to give care in the health field. We are going to have to begin, though, to bring into the health field people who are going to be more closely allied with it and who will, on a career basis, stay with it over a longer period of time.

So, as the whole world changes around us, we are even tripped up by the use of names. I think it is interesting, just as a problem in communication and learning, to see a nursing educator talk to a group of doctors and explain to them that this is general education and is not really closely related to activities in the hospital. Two or three weeks later, ask a group of doctors to give you the gist of what was said. They never remember the part that said that the hospital was no longer the central point in nurses' training.

But I think she has got a perfectly good point and I think we had better hear her. We are at the period of time when new professionals are going to have to be brought into the health field if the physician is to be able to discharge his duties. I would draw a parallel again with the nursing field. Some 20 years ago, I think it became obvious that there were not going to be enough nurses to carry out their function in the health field. But it was difficult to get this appreciated, and it was difficult to begin to put in programs which would eventually take up the slack in the nursing field.

The problem is highlighted to me by the fact that the nurse in our hospital is the only person who cannot learn. Now anybody else in the hospital can be upgraded in their work because they have time to learn something new every year. But our nurses have reached the point where they are in such short supply and are so overcome by their responsibilities that they frankly have no time for learning.

Now I think this is the same point that is beginning to confront the physician. If you watch the average physician in practice, you discover that he now has little time for learning. As we attempt to give medical care to the entire population, our current supply of physicians is not going to go around. Unless we begin to add more workers to the health field, the physician will find himself within the next 10 to 15 years in exactly the situation in which the nurse is. And for all I know, he may use the same solution: namely, withdraw as a major factor in the health field.

We do have a difference in point of view between those people who believe the past can be recreated and shored up by tinkering with it here or there, and those individuals who believe that a new era is beginning, an old era is ended, and that not too much time should be spent in tinkering with shoring up the past. It is clear that I believe one era is ended and another is started.

I would like to say just one word about the problem of putting doctors in relationship to people who haven't in the past received medical care. I was certainly a slow learner in this area. It is easy to learn something in one field and be not able to relate it to what your other hand is doing.

For years we have been concerned with the problem of what to do with people who have come from other countries with a much less well developed society than we have and a much less developed educational system than we have. Frequently they come to this country for college, where they spend four years. They go through four years of medical school. They then go through four or five years of professional training in this country. When they return home they find a society into which they cannot fit and find no niche in which they can be useful. Having made a large emotional commitment to one way of life, with 12 years of fairly hard work, they tend to be either unhappy where they are or tend to come back here.

We now wish to give modern medical care to a large section of our American citizenry who have received limited care in the past. We have the question of how do we get doctors to them. And it is becoming obvious to us that those bright black students who compete well in college, who get into the Harvard Medical School and who come to Duke for four years of postgraduate training are not of any help at all to us in this problem. And we are dealing with exactly the same kind of situation we were dealing with when we took other people out of their culture or changed the culture for 12 years and then wished them to go back to it.

In attempting to improve the ability of a doctor to give more services, we have begun to look at the question of how he should be supplied with assistants. We attempted to separate those things the physician does which require judgment from those which require some intelligence and some skill and which are recycled frequently every day. And, as you break down the activities of the physician in this way, it becomes obvious that many things which have been done traditionally by doctors can be done by non-doctors. We were also confronted with the fact that, at this time in history, specialization is with us, and that it is now very difficult for the hospital to produce a pool of personnel trained to fit the many needs of the various kinds and aspects of practice of medicine. It seemed to us that the physician had to define what his needs were, had to find that population which could serve those needs, and to train these people to act as his helpers.

We have begun to train a group of people we have elected to call physician's assistants, and that is exactly what they are. These are people who are recruited by the doctor; they are trained by the doctor and in the end we intend them to be paid by the doctor.

Of course, we have had the usual kind of problems which you would expect with any new area. We've had the question from nurses as to whether we were stealing things that belonged to them. We've had many questions from our own intern and resident staff and senior professional staff. Were we going to get in trouble by having people do things done traditionally by the physicians? Would the assistants eventually set up as doctors? We have had trouble from the hospital administrators who would like the command line to remain, through nursing service up to the hospital superintendent. They would like for the duties and the financial rewards of this particular group of people to be determined by hospital management rather than by doctors. We have had trouble with government in looking for support because they have said that, in order to work in the health field at any advanced level, you need a college degree. Having been to college myself, I've always been a little skeptical about this thesis. More than a college education, you need dedication to the health field and a willingness to give service, some understanding of why sick people are irrational and why they make demands that well people don't make.

Each year the physician's assistant can learn things he didn't know the year before. This has to be a lifetime commitment. He doesn't work a few years and stop, and a few years and stop, but says, "This is my business", and works at it year in and year out. In the men we have selected for training, the turn of the social wheel has been such that they have gone only through high school and are not financially in a position to go to college. I do not think we would gain anything by sending these men to four years of college, when they have identified that they want to be in the health field and are ready to go to work.

I am not advocating any particular thing except one, and that is I think the old system is ending and that we all ought to be trying out new programs which are possible to start in our own areas. I have talked about men and now I will say a few things about machines. As you know, this is a computerized era, and new ways to handle data are being brought to the health field.

As this type of machinery comes into being, one must continually re-examine the role of various people who are collecting the data and putting it into the machine. My own guess would be that a great deal of material that is characteristically collected by the physician can be collected by the non-physician and that this can be synthesized in the computer to the point at which the computer can begin to ask questions relevant to the patient's particular problem. And this is really the point at which medical practice is the easiest to teach and the easiest to learn. So we have this problem of computer-manpower interface, and what will the machine be like? What will the men be like? Obviously, we don't know yet.

The physician's assistant may want to become a doctor. If he does, he should be required to take the general education and the basic science courses required of the physician. His work as a physician's assistant could count towards the clinical training required of doctors. The amount of credit he could obtain would be determined by an appropriate examination. In practice, a physician's assistant with a family and a high school education will rarely become a physician. If one trained college graduates as assistants, a larger number would become doctors.

The point we come to immediately is that the physician has to be trained along with the physician's assistant; otherwise, he really doesn't know how to use him and know what to do with him. Our general plan was to have him have a year of didactic work, supervised by the people he is going to work with. The second year, we put the assistant in those areas of the hospital which have a high doctor-patient ratio. These include the emergency clinic, admitting room at the VA Hospital, recovery room, respiratory care unit, endocrine clinic, cardiac care unit, group and individual practices in North Carolina, State prison hospitals.

We hope to give our assistant an open-ended certificate and, indeed, this is what we are doing at the present time. The certificate states what we have taught him and what in our opinion he is able to do under the supervision of a doctor. Our terms of contract would be that whenever his doctor or doctors wanted him to do something which would be of benefit to the area in which he works, and for which he needs more training, we would train him. We then amend his certificate and say that now he is competent to do these additional procedures under the supervision of the doctor.

Most nurses, when they do work, work at jobs—as my wife works at a job—one which she can do and still take excellent care of me. Most of the nurses elect to work in areas such as the airport, where they are not heavily involved in the type of care needed in a busy hospital. I have no objection to this. I just come back to the fact that an awful lot of the work of the health field cannot be covered by this group.

The reason hospital-centered nurses cannot learn is that there are not enough of them. They cannot be released from the pressing duties of the day for new ventures. They cannot share in the continual learning process of the physician because of lack of time. The availability of time and learning are always related. If we were to have the number of interns drop below a certain level, all the learning would disappear. It takes time, irrespective of the service aspect, to master new kinds of material. And nurses just simply do not have the time in the day to be put aside for learning purposes.

And I think every profession can learn from this experience: that you cannot get too far behind in the manpower in the jobs you have agreed to cover without then getting into a situation in which you have extraordinarily little flexibility. I did not mean that an individual nurse, given the time to learn, was not able to learn. I meant that the system as now worked—at least in our part of the world—in which the numbers have become sufficiently low in regard to the tasks which have to be done—

there is no time to learn what you might like to the next year or the next year. [1967]

•

Nursing education at the degree level has become a form of general education and as such I am happy to support it. The girls are pretty and make fine wives.

As long as nurses insist that nursing has a different intellectual content from medicine, the matter cannot be resolved, and nurses will become increasingly less important in the health field. The nurse is either doing menial tasks or administration or practicing medicine. By tradition it is insisted that she cannot diagnose or treat patients. She is under a hierarchy which has a low ceiling and, if she breaks through the hierarchy and goes to a doctor to train her so that she can do more advanced diagnosis and treatment, she threatens the nursing leaders who have grown up with the old ceiling.

•

The faculty in nursing stressed the need for advanced degrees. These were usually taken in education or one of the social sciences. The net effect of this was that the members of the nursing faculty were usually less competent in dealing with sick patients than the average nurse. The more advanced the degree, the less capable one became at adding excitement to the clinical service.

* * * *

There are no two persons who are identical at a single point in time. Therefore, in the last analysis, every person belongs to his own subgroup. At the present state of our knowledge, we would gain nothing by attempting to write a complete description of each person. The differences which we know exist between two very similar persons who are functioning well in our society may not at this point in time be important enough to catalog. A subgroup which appears irrelevant at one time may be very relevant at another. For many years physicians carried Rh-positive and Rh-negative mothers in the same subgroup. In recent years we have learned that this is a mistake and we now subgroup them appropriately.

Persons have some subgrouping characteristics that last during a lifetime. As the body forms, matures, and ages, it is in continual interaction with its environment. Each interaction creates a difference which may be permanent or which may be reversible. Thus some subgrouping characteristics are transient, lasting only microseconds.

For the purpose of clinical practice, the physician recognized three primary types of subgroups:

1. The first type of subgroups are those to which patients belong during long periods of time and where the distinguishing characteristics are built into the system by genetic markers or by influences occurring before full maturation of the organism, such as hemophilia, congenital malformations due to rubella, alteration in the brain from malnutrition, fluoride impregnation of teeth, Marfan's syndrome, G-6-PD deficiency, differences in fingerprints.

2. The second type of subgroups are made up of persons exposed to an environmental stimulus of the required strength and timing to cause temporary or permanent change in the organism, for example, one of two identical twins may develop pneumonia. The exposure of one twin to the right combination of environmental influences, plus the right concentration of pneumococci, caused pneumonia. Disease imposed from the outside created a new subgroup for one of the twins. These subgroups created by environmental influences may be easily reversible, as in the cold; they may be made more reversible by treatment, as in the pneumococcal pneumonia; or they may last many years either with or without treatment, as in tuberculosis.

3. The third type of subgroups are produced by the interaction between permanent markers and environmental influences (physical stimuli, chemical interactions, or infection). The person with cystic fibrosis is unusually liable to infection; the man with multiple myeloma has more than his share of pneumococcal infection; the blind man has more problems with trauma; the person who makes peculiar or imperfect imprints in his central nervous system has more trouble with society.[5]

•

[*Technology Can Change Medical Practice*]: Though many thoughtful people believe that information sciences and technological changes induced by them will eventually revolutionize the practice of medicine, little change has actually occurred. At the practice interface, the doctor has discovered that he needs little information to practice medicine in the current modes. A list of the patient's problems (diagnoses), a summary of past diagnostic procedures, current medications, and a flowsheet of procedures to be done give him all the useful information that is usually available to him or to any of his colleagues. While this can be supplied by the computer, it is usually available to him in cheaper and equally useful formats. Computer-aided instruction is available to him, but journals, books, audiodigests, medical meetings and colleagues offer equally effective routes of education. There is nothing offered by the new approaches that is worth the trouble of overturning well-formed, lifelong patterns of practice and learning.

The technological revolution will come only when doctors or groups of doctors using computer technology have a clear advantage in practice over doctors who maintain the status quo. There is need for a careful delineation of an important problem that has no solution other than computerization.

Doctors in the practice of medicine collect a wide variety of information which allows them to make diagnoses. A diagnosis puts a patient into a subgroup of the population which is supposed to have a common outcome if untreated. Medical care is useful if it can favorably modify the course of patients who form this subgroup. The doctor may be useful if he determines that persons placed in a particular subgroup really do not have a common outcome. Many persons with a diagnosis of a potentially fatal illness can live a useful and unworried life if they can be informed that they are in a subgroup within the diagnostic category which does not have the morbidity and mortality characteristics usually associated with that particular diagnosis.

In actual practice, persons within a given diagnostic category (subgroup) may have widely different outcomes. A person with myocardial infarction may die in three minutes or live for 50-plus years. The doctor, therefore, on the basis of textbook, journal information and from his own experience, attempts to establish a few sub-categories under each diagnosis. The number he can carry in his head is small, and he is continually tricked by the capriciousness of his memory. If one watches him practice, one finds that the experiences of the last few months weigh unduly in his decision-making. One learns by experience that the behavior of any doctor is un-understandable unless the most recent inputs that affect his decision-making can be captured. Periodically he will be disturbed by his ignorance and, with great effort, will review the past experience of himself and his colleagues to determine the best treatment of a patient 60 years or older who has diabetes, myocardial infarction and aortostenosis. To his chagrin, he will discover that he has not established rigid criteria for any of the three diagnoses and that neither he nor his colleagues have the information which will allow him to determine whether the patients he is studying are a relatively homogeneous group with a predictable outcome or are a very heterogeneous group with widely differing outcomes. Fully knowing that he does not have good information, but urged on by the stimulus to give the best care to the next patient he sees with these diagnoses—and frequently by the desire to write a paper—he makes the assumption that these patients are a tight subgroup and he proceeds accordingly. He is neither better nor worse than any other doctor trying to describe the course of a chronic illness and endeavoring to give the patient good medical care.

An unusually compulsive doctor, collecting data on illnesses of short duration, will have better information on the course of the patients placed into a particular subgroup. But even here he is confronted with more subgroups than his memory can handle. He must deal with the disease from infancy to old age, from disease discovered early on the basis of symptoms to disease discovered by accident, from disease localized at discovery to disease generalized at discovery, from the process producing no disability to the process producing severe disability, from the disease producing no change beyond the first involved system to disease producing change in one or more than 20 subsystems, from disease occurring in genetically similar hosts to disease occurring in very genetically different hosts. It must come as no surprise that, with the exception of very acute processes, doctors are poor predictors of the course of illness, with or without treatment.

Computer science can change this picture. Information can be collected and stored in a way which allows the doctor to use all his experience to care for the patient—not just the portion he can remember. He can eventually use the total experience of his medical center and eventually that of other medical centers to care for his patients. The computer can carry many more subgroups in its memory than can the doctor. Only an examination of outcomes can determine the number of useful subgroups.

The Duke Medical Center has for the last five years been collecting a computerized data base to assist our doctors in caring for complex cardiovascular problems. Our first problem was to develop a data management team composed of doctors and computer scientists who were willing to make an investment in establishing a data bank which any doctor in practice in our institution could use. This data management group worked with experts in the cardiovascular field to define the descriptors to characterize the individual person. These descriptors are as close to the primary data as possible and are not a condensation of data into a conclusion or diagnosis. The statement that the changes in an electrocardiogram are diagnostic of myocardial infarction is not very helpful A description of the electrocardiogram is much more useful. The primary data remain useful even if the criteria for the diagnosis of myocardial infarction change over time or with a new set of doctors. The descriptors of the patient population will change over time. Many will be found to be useless. Medical science will demonstrate the need for new ones.

The data management team had to convince the doctors that the data collected from the patients belonged to the institution and not to them. This meant that there had to be agreement on definitions and that all the data had to be stored in a central file. The doctor had to give up his prerogative of storing parts of the data in his private file and changing the data whenever he felt that new information made his previous grouping erroneous. The doctors had to accept the fact that the data management section would not process data to build the bank unless it was validated and that, in many instances, non-physician personnel would be better validators than the doctors themselves.

The traditional functions of storing, clustering the data and retrieving the data have presented an interesting series of problems, but they are not nearly as difficult as the problems of collecting validated data for input into the system. Collection of a proper data base cannot be piggy-backed onto practice. The creation of the data base is expensive. The doctor in practice can use the data base, and this expense can be borne by patient care funds. The development of the data base and its extension by data from new patients is expensive, and every doctor using the data base cannot contribute new data to the base.

The use of the data base is based on the fact that we are matching our patient with patients who are enough like him to have a similar course either treated or untreated. This means that both short-term and long-term outcomes must be known. This adds a new dimension to medical practice because the knowledge of outcomes of similar patients becomes an essential part of the data bank. This is an expensive but necessary part of the system.

We are far enough along to begin to feel the power of the data bank. We intend to reach the point where no clinical decisions will be made on the care of any patient with coronary artery disease, myocardial infarction or heart block until the data bank has been searched and the outcomes of similar patients have been given to the doctor. When the Duke Medical Center can bring immediately all its experience to bear on each cardiovascular patient entering its doors, it will have a clear lead over all other doctors. It will be in the position of those departments of pathology which began to use electron, phase and fluorescent microscopy. Other pathologists hated to learn the new way but, to remain competitive, they had to use the new tools.

Once the problem has been cracked in a major area in a single medical center, progress will be rapid. Patient care funds will be a better financial resource, because the care given by the updaters and users of the data bank will be of superior quality. The greatest profits from the system will accrue when several medical centers begin to pool their data. At the present time there is not enough incentive for different medical centers to reach common definitions, common methods of validating data, and a common method for storage and retrieval. When one medical center has established the system, there will be a strong incentive for other centers to put their house in order and join the system.

We are also pushed to implement an adequate system for describing and more accurately subgrouping patients by the amount of public money being expended to evaluate therapeutic procedures in chronic illness. Patients with a common diagnosis are commonly randomized into two groups: one treated and one not treated. The statisticians erroneously believe that patients with a given diagnosis are a homogeneous subgroup and, untreated, will have a common outcome. Nothing can be further from the truth. Patients given the diagnosis of coronary arterial disease are not a homogeneous group. No one knows how many subgroups would have to be defined to select persons who run a reasonably common course. My own guess would be one hundred. No single institution can produce enough patients to define all the clinically useful subgroups. In desperation, all the patients are considered to be alike and some therapeutic intervention is started. The intervention may cause great harm to some, not affect others, and help some. The study predictably comes out with no sharp answer except for the bill of many millions of dollars.

Chronic, multifactorial disease problems can be studied, but not by the methods of the present or past. If one wishes to create useful information on which to base therapeutic trials, computer technology must be exploited.

In summary, major technological changes will not occur in medical schools until this technology can accomplish worthwhile results which give the practitioner using these tools an advantage over his competitors. Therapeutic trials in chronic illness cannot be meaningful until better ways to form tighter subgroups who run a uniform course are operational. Duke Medical Center has identified the area where the leverage lies, and has a five-year investment in preparing for the new day. [1972]

•

[*Information and Chronic Illness*]: A great deal of thought and effort have gone into structuring systems which will make available to the biomedical investigator the data created by the scientists of the world. We know that the investigator who has easy access to information from the past and a way to tap the flow of current information has a great advantage over the person with more limited access to these sources. We have established an extensive library system throughout the world to make data from the past available, and the International Research Communication System is a fine example of our successful efforts to make current information available and useful.

The practicing physician has a great need for an information system to be developed which is useful in the care of individual patients with chronic illness. Every new patient who presents himself to the doctor with a major chronic illness should be regarded by the doctor as a research problem. This is an impossible approach with our present information system. One has to spend many hours of time in the library attempting to identify patients with known outcomes who are like the current patients, and the odds are that he will not find a single one. Doctors have never created a system where the descriptors of the new patient can be used to look up patients with like descriptors who have been followed for years until the final outcome is known. Patients with chronic disease will have many forms of treatment. Each form of treatment is simply another descriptor. The difficulty is that, in chronic illness, the doctor does not know the outcome of patients treated or untreated. The doctor cannot tell the patient exactly what medicine has to offer him or the expected morbidity and expense of different forms of treatment.

The problem is a formidable one because chronic illness by definition lasts many years, and the doctor may see the patient in the first year or in the thirtieth year of the process. Because of the length of the illness, many changes not related to the disease, as well as changes related to the disease, will occur and the descriptors of the patient at any point should include enough information to accurately characterize the patient.

How many descriptors does one need, and how does he know that he has the right descriptors? This answer cannot be given in advance. The doctor needs to know what descriptors characterize patients who reach an agreed-upon endpoint. There has to be a constant feedback of information between outcomes which indicate the actual degree of homogeneity of the sub-groups supposedly made homogeneous by the selection of common descriptors and the doctor who selects and records the descriptors.

There are several reasons why a doctor does not have at his disposal a data bank arranged in dictionary form, with descriptors characterizing patients who have similar outcomes.

1. The medical profession is not accustomed to collecting precise data because it has had no place to store it and no ability to retrieve it. The doctor can carry in his head the information he needs to care for an acute episode in a patient with chronic illness. He has no way to use any data to focus on long-term goals.

2. There has been no demonstration that the doctor with a data base at his disposal can practice better medicine than a doctor without this information.

3. Medical centers support short-term projects and are unable to fund a new program that requires a number of years of hard work before the program produces demonstrable results.

4. Clinical data banks have not been institutionalized. They can be turned on or off as investigators move or money becomes scarce. They do not have the stability of the university library.

5. Medical centers have not established clinical data banking as a profession. Investigators collect data to perform experiments and they discard data not applicable to the experiment. A data banker collects data to determine the homogeneity of his subgroups. All data are grist for his mill.

6. Computer technology is just now developing to the point where the doctor in practice can easily tap the data bank.

7. There must be a long lead period between the collection of the original patients and the determination of the homogeneity of the groups as defined by outcomes. There will be a period of at least two years—and more commonly, four years—before the doctors collecting the data begin to have a return for their efforts.

We know that in time doctors will give up diagnosis as we now know it. They will determine the descriptors which will adequately describe the biological, social and economic measurements of the new patient. The computer will search through millions of records of patients with known outcomes and will give the doctor the data on patients like the one he has just described. The skill of the doctor will lie in his ability to select and record the correct descriptors.

The material in the bank becomes more useful when the information can be stored as it is gathered. For example, the measurements characterizing the electrocardiogram are more useful than the doctor's interpretation of the electrocardiogram. The measurements from the x-ray of the chest are more useful than the interpretation of the x-ray. The building of the clinical data bank forces the doctor to have a greater interest in developing an appropriate engineering interface so that the biologic data can be quantitated and stored more effectively.

The description of the patient in the computer bank needs to be broader than the diagnosis that the doctor is accustomed to use to indicate the state of the patient. Economic, social and cultural features have a significant effect on outcomes. The patient needs to know what medicine has to offer him and at what cost in terms of complications, morbidity, mortality and expense. No patient with a chronic problem can find this out at present because no doctor knows.

Regardless of the progress made in prevention of disease, persons will eventually develop chronic problems that require medical care. At the present, and in the foreseeable future, immense sums of money will be spent at this interface. A great deal will be wasted, because the doctor always tries. He has no way to know when his efforts are really useful. A clinical computer bank will be expensive, but not as expensive as our system of care which at present cannot be evaluated. [1973]

•

The question as to whether the information in the data bank would be accepted and used by the doctor in practice is a very important one.

The material in the data bank is of the same kind and quality that the doctor practicing medicine has used throughout his professional life. Instead of turning to textbooks, monographs, journals or colleagues to find out how patients have responded in the past, he turns to the computer. The information is on line and within a few minutes he has the material that would have taken many months to extract from the library. Because of the large storage capacity of the computer, he can have precise data on a large number of patients who are most nearly like his current patient and, because the description of each patient is coupled to followup, he can have outcome data on a large number of patients like his new patient.

The doctors interested in clinical research will use the computer bank in the same way that they now use the hospital record room. Doctors interested in therapeutic trials can identify from the data bank the characteristics of patients who come to common endpoints, and can determine if a given treatment causes patients to come to a better endpoint.

The data bank can be a very useful tool, but it is only that. It is a mechanical physician's assistant. It is not the doctor. It will not help with management of a particular patient who is restricted in diet, activity, and the use of medications by religious beliefs. Such problems are the province of the doctor and cannot be usurped by computers.

I do believe that the doctor will sharpen and make more quantitative his clinical information when he knows that his observations will be available for daily use and not buried in the hospital record room.

•

I believe the developments in the information field are going to have the greatest impact on medical education in the next generation, and Duke has developed a rather considerable lead in this area. One of my close friends started in the information area in his bank 25 years ago. He rapidly rose to the rank of vice president. I asked him if he wanted to be president. He said that he couldn't care less. He controlled the computerized information system, and the bank could not operate without him. Under those circumstances, he held the real power no matter who had the titles.

In essence, we have coupled a detailed description of each patient and his treatment, with followup of the patient until his death. Our followup is better than 99%. Our doctors now treat each new patient with coronary disease as a research patient. Once the new patient is described, we can within minutes tell the doctor what has happened to like patients treated in different ways. This gives the doctor for the first time a way to combine diagnosis with prognosis. He has information of a kind never before available to him to help in his decision-making process. [1976]

* * * *

[*Why Moon Walking Is Simpler Than Social Progress*]: On May 25, 1961, President Kennedy announced that the United States would land a man safely on the moon before 1970. The resources of the nation were mobilized and the goal of moon walking was met. Many thoughtful people in this country are puzzled by the fact that we can undertake a project of this magnitude and yet have no solution for poverty, ignorance, prejudice, greed, racism and war. They declare that a country which can produce a moon stroll on schedule can solve the important social problems on this earth if it tries hard enough. They believe that our major social problems can be solved a) by redirecting toward selected social goals the flow of funds now committed to the Vietnam war and to space exploration, and b) by redirecting toward the solution of defined social problems the energies of the scientists and engineers now working in defense and space. Thoughtful analysis of the problem will make it clear why the brilliant performances in space or defense do not lead to increased competence in preventing poverty, prejudice and pillage.

Given adequate financial support, the nation could meet its moon goal because:

1) It was not necessary to involve all the population. One could select and choose those human beings with the necessary talents and the desire to take part in the venture.

2) The object to be built was inanimate and inanimate objects do not arouse intense feelings. Therefore, people of widely different cultures, educational backgrounds and beliefs could be mobilized to work on the space project.

3) It was possible and practical to change the design and construction of the rocket whenever the structure underway was found not to assure a functioning space ship. Any faulty part could be replaced at will. Initial errors could be corrected.

How different is the situation when man is the machine to be made! The prevention of ignorance, poverty, racism, prejudice and war depend on the accurate design and proper construction of human machines which will function to produce a society of intelligent, constructive and tolerant men. Man is made from the union of the egg and sperm. If certain elements are missing from the genetic material which programs the system, development of this human organism into an optimally functioning person is impossible. We will forever, until the organism dies, be dealing with an imperfect instrument. We cannot replace the defective parts and construct a better design.

As the fertilized egg develops, it is highly sensitive to environmental influences which at critical times can cause permanent changes in the final machine. A drug may inhibit development of a limb bud, or rubella virus may cause minor or major defects. At birth, the nervous system is still remarkably plastic. Favorable environmental influences will favor developments useful to society; unfavorable influences will favor changes that will be detrimental to society.

In the early years, many of the changes in the nervous system produced by the interplay between hereditary and environmental influences are easily reversible. There are, however, no provisions for replacement of injured or sick nervous cells by new and viable nerve cells. The cells of the nervous system must last throughout the lifetime of the organism. The reversibility in the adult nervous system results from molecular changes within existing nerve cells, not from the addition of new cells. After the age of six, more and more of the final structure is fixed, and a smaller and smaller portion of the total structure contains reversible elements. In the early years, a child can learn several languages without conscious effort. He can speak each one with the native's accent. After the age of six, the nervous system loses this ability to accept alteration from the environment without effort. Any language learned thereafter will require effort. Learning does not occur in a vacuum. Anything retained in the nervous system requires an alteration in the molecular structure of the nervous system. Any unlearning requires a change in structure. The older we become the greater must be the energy input to produce any change in structure.

The child grows and matures with his nervous system becoming more fixed each year. There is no way to redesign or replace poorly developed portions of his nervous system. Fears, hates, prejudices and poor patterns of learning and performance become permanent parts of the system. It is important to remember that prejudices and other feelings are produced by finite changes in the structure of the nervous system. They are a manifestation of molecular arrangement—not of mysticism. They cannot be altered unless one can alter nerve cells at the molecular level.

When our nation faces its social problems today, we have the problem of building a rational, cohesive society out of a series of twisted and tortured components. We have to live with what we have grown, and we have no knowledge of how to alter, to a sufficient degree to guarantee social progress, what we have grown.

It is clear that we must continue our search for knowledge for many years before we shall know how to modify the genetic and environmental factors to allow production of men who can live together in peace. Even the thought of genetic and environmental manipulations which would produce men without our present cultural characteristics and built-in prejudices frightens mankind. Peoples' feelings about people are quite different from peoples' feelings about non-human machines.

If one believes that man is a free agent who can alter the structure of his nervous system at any time by the exercise of free will, one can be optimistic about rapid social progress. If, on the other hand, one believes that an adult man is a machine whose structure has in it a limited number of reversible elements, one must be much more pessimistic about rapid social progress. This is the answer to the question of why a nation which can send a man to the moon has no easy solution for the social problems of this earth.

As man begins to regard himself in a more natural way, he appreciates that he is in reality a machine which must operate within well-defined limits tightly bound by his structure. As he understands the growth and development of his nervous system, he will devote more energy to the health of the mothers producing the man-machine which sets the limits of social progress. He will use a larger portion of his resources to affect favorably the development of this man-machine during its early and more plastic years. He will pay more attention to the development of the structural changes which express themselves as feelings and lead man to destroy man.

It is important at this time that decision makers creating public policy understand what we must do if we wish to be able to modify man's relationship to man. Agencies designed to have an effect on social systems must be structured and programmed in an entirely different fashion from those which can produce superb engineering feats. Excellence in one area by no means assures excellence in another.[6]

•

Most people are idealistic when they're young; even *I* used to vote for liberal things.

•

In uncommon diseases one must think more in uncommon references. All too often the older physician looks at older frames of reference.[7]

•

Very little money is spent for research and development on systems which can bring together the many subsystems necessary for a health care delivery system. Money is spent for the development of specific items which can be purchased by any of the purveyors of health care. Larger sums would be required to implement the necessary mix of men and machines to make major innovations and put modern technology to work to serve entire cities, groups of cities or regions. Private industry does not believe there is a market for the sale of such systems and is not developing them.

One of the difficulties is in our account system. Industry counts as profits only dollars. An instrument which saves the life of 1,000 mothers may cost five million dollars to develop. The potential market is only 1,000, and the developmental costs cannot be justified by private industry. The fact that the 1,000 mothers raised their children, kept their families together, and made important contributions to the nation will not appear in the accounting. Therefore the instrument is not produced. [1976]

•

The only solution I've ever seen to poverty is more money.

•

I have the same difficulty as you in separating health maintenance from housing, food, transportation, recreation and education. I have gradually lost my faith in the ability of the capitalistic system to meet these needs unless it is modified in some way so that each person will make a greater contribution to society.

In the past we have tried to meet major human needs by obtaining money from private sources or from taxes. Philanthropy cannot possibly supply the needed funds. I do not believe the middle-aged to elderly persons who have the majority of the funds in the nation will agree to be taxed sufficiently to allow our survival as a nation. Some other device must be found.

National service for a two-year period for every young man and woman is a possible solution. Our society enriches our lives in many ways. Each will have to give more to the society if we want to reap these benefits. We must have the labor force to rebuild our cities, control our pollution, produce our houses and feed our people. Young people will give of themselves more than old people will give of their money.

I am aware that Hitler turned to this device and used it for poor ends. Theoretically, any method may be used for good or for bad ends. [1969]

REFERENCES

1. Stead EA, contributor. IN The Future of Medical Education. Duke University Press, Durham, 1973.
2. Stead EA. New England J. Med. **277**: 800, 1967.
3. Stead EA. Medical Times **97**: 246, 1969.
4. Stead EA. Ann. Int. Med. **72**: 271, 1970.
5. Stead EA. Arch. Int. Med. **127**: 703, 1971.
6. Stead EA. Medical Times **97**: 248, 1969.
7. Schoonmaker F, Metz E. Just Say For Me. World Press Inc., Denver, 1968.

Now Having Had My Say, Blessings on You

MANY PETITIONED EAS FOR ADVICE

[*To a prospective visiting professor*]: I want to remind you again that your time as speaker on October 24 is limited. In my experience, most people with a broad subject and a limited time do one of two things: either they say nothing at all, which is certainly bad, or they say so many things that the audience goes home not knowing what was said, which is equally bad. The only alternative is to select a few things which you think are really worth remembering and then say each one of them over three times. It is preferable that you not say them with the same words, but there is no doubt that the repetition is essential. Your letter frightens me only because it means you are going to fall into the second of the traps I mentioned above. *Now, having had my say, blessings on you and do what you want to.*

•

[*To a former colleague at Emory*]: You certainly have a knotty problem. Somebody has to accept the responsibility for training Negro physicians, and this responsibility, of course, entails undergraduate and postgraduate work. When one considers the need for graduate training, particularly hospital training, it is difficult to see how one can avoid turning the Negro section of Grady over to Negro interns. It will still be a considerable number of years before Negro physicians can work in any numbers on the white wards and clinic without conflict.

The University can assume the responsibility for training these Negro doctors. If it does so, it will most certainly wish to go into undergraduate training of Negroes, being driven there by the present inadequacies of this training. This really means a doubling of the student body and, in effect, the operation of two medical schools. The other alternative is to cooperate as much as possible in the program of graduate training of Negro physicians, but to insist that the state, city or federal governments assume the actual responsibility and supply the staff.

My own feeling is that this is a state responsibility, and that Emory

Medical School would do well to give it to them. I say this because it will be a number of years before the teaching of these men will be sufficiently interesting to hold the attention of your present faculty. I do not think the immediate presence of a few Negro interns working at Grady would alter the picture, but I see no way to keep these few from becoming many. This, of course, does not alter your relationships with the rest of Grady Hospital except insomuch as your financial holds on the Hospital Authority are in the colored units. I certainly have always felt that university planning should not block the eventual use of the Negro service at Grady Hospital for the training of Negro physicians. I know of no other way in which the health problem in the South can be approached and, as you know, a situation of this kind is one of the few valid arguments for the socialization of medicine. I think the points to be stressed are that taking on this new group of doctors for training requires new personnel and additional financial support regardless of what method is used. [1950]

•

[*To a colleague*]: I happened to review your record on . . . and note that you use the terms hematuria and hemaglobinuria interchangeably. As you undoubtedly know, on reflection these are not the same thing. I am merely taking the trouble to call this to your attention on the general thesis that your friends will take time to correct your mistakes while the less friendly folk will ignore you.

•

I sincerely regret that I am unable to remember you and for this reason could not write a convincing recommendation. I would suggest that you use the name of someone more familiar with your recent work. I am sorry for my poor memory and trust this has not delayed you unduly.

•

[*To a public health official*]:   My own experience has been that it is difficult to interest people in health matters when they are well, and that any public education which goes toward arousing people and making them think in health terms is beneficial. I do not doubt that polio has raised money out of proportion to the death rate from that disease. As a byproduct of their work, though, education in all health fields has improved.

The situation is somewhat analogous to that in the school system. Through a survey of elementary education in the state, one could logically object to the expenditure of funds for the University of North Carolina, because the University touches only a few people while elementary education in many areas is very poor. However, I do not think that is sound thinking. By making the University good, one learns what education can actually accomplish and this eventually has a direct and forceful effect on the elementary system.

•

[*To the Duke Medical School Dean*]: In Executive Committee on Friday, I voiced my disappointment over the methods of procedure of the committee charged with planning for the future of psychiatry in the medical school.

Our collective background of psychiatry is founded in the experience of the Hopkins group with Adolf Meyer. He was an unfathomable mystery to generations of Hopkins students and men trained in those years looked on psychiatry as apart from the mainstream of medicine. In the years at Duke, we have had no leaders in the field of psychiatry education and, to a large extent, the department has remained a subject for joking and ridicule. I have listened to many stories told over the last five years in Executive Committee meetings which have illustrated the general attitude.

During the last 10 years, university departments of psychiatry have developed which are contributing richly to the training of students, residents and senior staff. To my knowledge, none of the members of our Executive Committee has spent as much as a week in these new centers. Experience by faculty members of the success of these programs would allow us to know how important a place in the educational sun is deserved by psychiatry.

In my opinion, psychiatry will be the most important single discipline in the medical schools of the next generation. I had hoped that the committee would bring to the Executive Committee a present-day evaluation of psychiatry in medical education. If my estimate of its importance is correct, the committee should present a strong argument to the Executive Committee to expand our facilities for psychiatry. If it is incorrect, I would like to have the committee present its evidence for its conclusions.

I think that our greatest need at the present moment is to clearly determine what psychiatry can contribute to us. Before that is done, we are not in position to plan for the future. [1952]

•

[*To colleagues who had inquired about a speaker being a windbag*]: I was out of town when . . . spoke here, but the consensus in the department indicates that there is no reason why you should change your mind about him as a speaker.

•

[*To another chairman of Medicine who questioned the value of assigning house staff to private wards*]: We do assign interns, assistant residents and clinical clerks to our private service. We have teaching rounds four days per week from 10:00 A.M. to 12:00. These are the usual type of bedside rounds. Sometimes the patients are being cared for by the rounding man and sometimes they are patients of other staff men.

This program is a troublesome one. The house staff do not obtain the same emotional satisfaction as they do from the ward patients. The patient knows that he is paying the staff physician, and he looks to him for final decisions.

In the long run, though, the program is worth its trouble. The students and house staff do see the kind of problems that they will handle in practice. They are forced to take care of patients rather than diseases.

The program is useful as a part of the student's and intern's experience. It is not a substitute for the public ward service and outpatient clinic.

•

[*To a colleague who has praised a paper by Dr. Stead*]: I am not sure how to use the word "creative". All the ideas which have been credited to me can be found somewhere in the writings and thoughts of others. My own contribution has been to realize that these particular notions were important and to design appropriate experiments to demonstrate their importance. We know that in most biological problems we are dealing with systems of multiple variables. Studying nearly any one of these intensively and setting up situations where one of the variables has a more dominant role nearly always gives additional information as to the latent possibilities of the system.

•

[*To a Public Health Official*]: I am not certain what information you want in regard to the sale of dietary ice cream and beverage drinks. In the practice of medicine, we do have need for our patients to be able to purchase a wide variety of foods. We are frequently interested in dairy products which contain a minimal amount of fat, as well as in beverage drinks which are low in calories. My own belief would be that careful and accurate labeling is of utmost importance. I believe many foods should be available which would not normally be fed to children but which are very useful in the treatment of older people; for example, in many of our problems, we would very much like to prescribe cheese which is of lower fat content than is now available; for other patients, it would be desirable to have cheese of a high fat content. What we need is both types, clearly labeled. [1957]

•

[*To a colleague approaching retirement*]: My chief personal contacts with you over the years have been in watching you work with medical students and house staff. I have admired the wisdom shown by you as you have handled the problems handed to you. Even more, I have been impressed by the sparkle in the eyes of the students and staff as they have thought with you. You freely give of yourself and they freely respond.

You have made your mark in the areas of patient care, research and teaching. You combine them in a way that makes all three into one whole. In this synthesis lies some of the secret of your ability to inspire others.

We admire your personal charm, your many talents and your devotion to the best ideals in medicine. May the years continue to treat you kindly.

•

[*Tribute to colleague receiving an honorary doctorate at Duke*]: Your career as a scientist and educator has been a distinguished one. These achievements brought to you the opportunity to become director of the National Institutes of Health at a time when major decisions in policy were being made. Under your guidance the National Institutes have become a dominant force in all research activities in the health fields. The number and quality of papers appearing on the programs of the learned societies demonstrate the scientific success of the Institutes. The opportunity to bring to bear on biological problems all the disciplines of basic science has been fully utilized. There has been a free flow of men between the Institutes and the universities. An increasing number of our faculty are alumni of yours, and an increasing number of our young men are looking to you for a portion of their training. The Institutes of Health, which might have become a white elephant, have become the strongest single force in the biological world. [1958]

•

[*To a colleague*]: I am not in agreement with the recommendation that an Institute of Gerontology be established within the National Institutes of Health. It would seem to me that, from the administrative point of view, the multiplicity of institutes is going to have to stop. Gerontology cuts across every conceivable branch of learning. I think there should be an administrative area within the NIH where the problems directly related to gerontology could be concentrated and the program given the necessary administrative impetus, but I do not believe that this requires the creation of a separate institute. [1958]

•

[*Arbitrating differences among colleagues*]:

a. I think he is a difficult person with a grudge against the world, and I would not trust his judgment on any complex matter. I regret that we have a bad apple in the barrel. . . .

b. I am sorry you and . . . became crossed up. Since I have the utmost respect for both of you, I will not take sides in this argument. You are different kinds of people, and this explains why you are doing the kind of medicine you are and why . . . is a fine neurologist. I know that the intentions of both of you are to give the best of medical care.

•

[*To a former resident*]:   I would not take a formal degree in education. To some degree, they are always rediscovering the wheel.

•

I think we don't have any real need for a senior-senior society. We all are free to go to the meetings of the present Southern Society, and I should think we all now make enough administrative decisions without being involved in a new set of them. I therefore vote "no" on this proposal. [1960]

•

[*To colleague who recommended accepting drug company funds*]: I have talked with a number of folk in the department and the general feeling is that they prefer not to have a party supported by the drug companies. I confess that these lines become a little blurred in my mind. I am sure that a portion of the money contributed by individual departments would come from drug house sources. I have some question in my own mind as to whether the departments should put up funds for supporting a party. I personally would rather contribute departmental funds toward getting one or two physicians from other countries to the meeting. Having grown up in an era when salaries were much lower and in which travel expenses to meetings were never paid, I cannot help thinking that the present generation can buy the drinks it needs. [1960]

•

[*Reply to a request for a contribution*]:   Somewhat to the surprise of both you and me, I'm going to say no to your request. The demands made on our family for support of various named professorships have reached the breaking point. I could not be comfortable in the role of sponsor unless I were prepared to make a substantial personal contribution.

As you know, the Thorndike with its staff was one of the most important experiences of my life. I was and am a great admirer of . . . and I will try to pass on to other generations of students the things which he taught me. This will have to be my memorial to him.

•

[*To officer of the American Society for Clinical Investigation*]:

a) With the present limit on membership, too many capable men are denied membership. The rejected candidates are too like the accepted ones, and the feeling exists that personal preference rather than scientific merit has been the deciding factor.

Clinical investigation must by its definition begin in the clinic where sick patients, students and staff meet and formulate problems. The development of the clinician and the seeing of the sick are time-consuming. The men who assume the traditional responsibilities of teaching, research and patient care will produce fewer purely laboratory studies than men in research institutes. It makes little difference whether those research institutes are located at the National Institutes of Health, the Rockefeller Institute, or are sequestered away in a medical school. Unless the Society can accommodate the leaders in medical departments who are concerned with the care of the ill, those same professors of medicine who for many years have supported the Society must begin to devalue it and turn elsewhere, either to a new society or to the narrower specialty societies. [1961]

b) Since you have already included his name in the booklet, let's let the matter stand. I had decided to withdraw his nomination because it was obvious that the members of the Council did not recognize the sterling values in him which are so well known at Duke. As I have said before, it is hard for a generalist to survive in current academic circles, even though most of us know that intellectually these people make a tremendous contribution. I guess the problem is that, knowing . . . to be a pearl of great price, I hesitate to put him up for a longer exposure into the too-rarified atmosphere. As you can tell, he is a person who will not be influenced unduly either by selection or rejection by our Society.

•

[*An intern from another school has asked that he be released from a Duke residency commitment*]:

a) We are not in a position to release you from your contract unless we have a satisfactory replacement. At this time of year it seems unlikely that we will. The decision as to whether you honor your own contract is purely a personal one, and I think this matter will have to be left entirely in your hands.

b) Your letter of March 2 closes out our relationship. I think, to protect others, I will write to your dean in order to have this made part of your record.

c) Dr...., who graduated from your school in June . . ., accepted a place with us on the medical house staff for July. He has now seen fit to break this contract with us and I think you should be familiar with this. This is the first instance we have had of this kind among your graduates. For the protection of other people, I think this should be made part of his record.

•

[*To referring M.D.s upset by residents at the "ivory tower"*]: a) The question of criticism about referring physicians is a difficult one. We make every effort to avoid it. We make too many mistakes of our own to enjoy throwing stones at anyone. By the very nature of our being a referral center, we do have many patients who are highly critical of the medical profession. They bring us very unlikely tales about their doctor and carry home very unlikely tales about us.

b) I appreciate your reluctance to state names and persons, but we do make more progress when specific instances are reported to us and we have the opportunity to use the incident as a mechanism for learning. We never use the troubles of any staff member for destructive purposes, because we always find that the heart was in the right place but that, for the moment, the brain failed.

•

[*Response to a Duke Parking Ticket*]: I am enclosing $1 to cover Duke University traffic violation charge No. 4911. I do not wish to argue the matter and will list this $1 as a contribution.

•

[*Advising a former resident that "Life is hard"*]: The difficulty in problems such as yours usually involves failure to make the compromises necessary to make the system work.

•

[*Recommendation to NIH*]: While I have no reservations about supporting the man, I am less enthusiastic about his current project. Because of his background, he is not very knowledgeable about medical affairs, and he is putting undue emphasis on the problem of the problem-oriented medical record. In due time, he will discover that the form of the record is not very important. The accuracy of the information in the record is the important consideration. Once the data are in, the computer can output them in a variety of forms.

The proposal he submitted is naive in that he believes doctors are very stirred up about the problem-oriented record. In actuality, doctors worry about records only when changes are made that touch their pocketbooks.

•

[*To former resident*]: I'm afraid that there is a penalty for strong arousal of feeling states, regardless of the right and wrong. I've gently tested the local waters and do not believe any good would be done by my bringing your name forcefully to the Carolina folk. I'm not judging the validity of the feelings: I'm merely recognizing their existence.

•

[*To a colleague desiring membership in the Association of American Physicians*]: The Association, in its mind's eye, represents a club which brings together all disciplines for consideration of problems related to human disease. In actual fact, it is a club of internists.

Most of the time, the non-career internist discovers that he cannot find the time to attend the more general meetings of the Association. Therefore, there is a tendency for the Council not to elect deans and persons strongly identified with a specialty.

This is a very low-key organization which does nothing but run an annual meeting. Don't take us very seriously.

•

[*To the Duke Dean who had asked for help re. a record librarian's complaint*]: The abbreviation "SOB" for shortness of breath is in nation-wide use, and we will be unable to stop its appearing in the Duke records.

•

[*To a foreign medical school*]: Your new school, your wide adminis-trative responsibilities and your past record of performance all tempt me to break my traditions and look beyond the States. In my dreams I accept, but in the cold light of day I know I had better stay home and work where I know the people and the culture.

•

[*To an organization requesting data*]: In my opinion, questionnaires of this type are worthless. One mixes good observations with poor ones. When the data are assembled in tables and published, the fact that it is junk escapes the reader. We have just gone through a national catastrophe because of this type of activity. Inaccurate and accurate data from Vietnam were mixed together. This tremendous collection of data went through successive distillations and was assembled into ever more impressive tables. This material was finally fed to the generals and the President, who fought a long war with little accurate information. [1974]

•

[*Lessons from Dr. Stead's China trip*]: I am not one who believes in a one-class health system any more than I believe in one type of grocery store or one type of automobile or sailing ship. China does have a one-class medical system. It also has a one-class system for all other human needs. I enjoyed my visit to China but have no desire to join up. [1975]

•

[*To the dean of another school*]: Just one word of philosophy: specializa-tion remains the cutting edge of scientific medicine. When any family practitioner wishes to further his knowledge of biology and illness, he does not go to another practitioner. He goes to the specialist. Without a strong core of specialists in medicine, gynecology, obstetrics, and pediatrics, your family practitioners will wilt on the vine. The specialist in the above disciplines cannot function without specialized and skilled surgeons.

I appreciated that family practitioners have attempted to increase their competence by a heavier investment in the social sciences. When the chips are down, these disciplines play little part in the daily work of the doctor. The nurses tried the same ploy and failed.

You need a strong department of medicine. The chief should be sympathetic to family medicine, but his primary responsibility is the development of excellence in the department of medicine. [1975]

•

[*To an investigator who is a frustrated member of a board of directors*]: The only way to get more dollars for research is to fix the percentage; then you will still lose because . . . will squirm out by changing the definition of research. Then we'll have to have meetings to determine definitions. Still, he will win because he has more time. [1975]

•

[*To a young faculty member following his initial encounter with Dr. Stead*]: The house staff will learn a great deal because of the interplay between you and me. They tend to be involved in the technical aspects of medicine and rarely consider the overall problem of patient care. They need to be jarred out of their common framework of reference, and the two of us did it. These types of problems usually involve the sacrifice of someone's ego. In this case it was yours. Next time around, I will be the sacrificial goat.

I thought you handled yourself superbly. I'm glad that you have risen to my level of consciousness. I also hope you will know who I am as we pass in the corridors. [1976]

•

[*To a former patient*]: After careful consideration of your case history, I have concluded that I have done everything I can do for you within my field of medical practice, and that further consultation with me would only involve needless expenditure of money for you. Therefore, I am requesting that you not attempt to make further appointments with me either through the Medical Private Diagnostic Clinic or otherwise.

Upon your request and authorization, I will make available to any physician information regarding the diagnosis and treatment you have received from me. [1966]

8

When the Heart Cannot Perform Its Task

EXCERPTS FROM MEDICAL PAPERS

Congestive heart failure occurs *when the heart cannot perform its task* of moving blood forward. It is the end result of many different pathologic processes which range from genetic defects through mechanical trauma. When the heart no longer performs adequately its role as a pump, the organs of the body are less well perfused. As blood accumulates in the venous systems of the lesser and greater circulations, organs are less well drained. The fall in cardiac output, the decreased blood supply to all organs, the congestion of all organs, and the redistribution of blood lead to many extensive changes in function of all the cells and organs of the body.

•

I have been interested in congestive heart failure since the beginning of my third year in medical school. The time was 1930, 39 years ago. In those days Soma Weiss and Tinsley Harrison were our gods. They drew the necessary distinction between heart disease, a pathologic process, and heart failure, a physiologic disturbance resonating through the entire body when one or both ventricles are unable to pump blood in a normal fashion. These men worked out the changes which occur in the lungs in acute left ventricular failure and they were well aware that severe left ventricular failure occurs in the presence of a normal systemic venous pressure. Both of these giants were interested in the nervous system and they knew that many of the physiologic changes produced by heart failure are dependent on an intact and reactive nervous system. They both emphasized that at any one given level of heart failure the intensity of the complaining is a function of the nervous system.

In the early 1940s, measurement of the cardiac output by right heart catheterization was popularized and the presence or absence of heart failure could be determined by measuring the cardiac output, the distribution of blood between the arterial and venous systems, and the flow of blood to the organs of the body. Heart failure is present when the heart, because of heart disease, cannot maintain the normal flow of blood to organs and cannot maintain the normal distribution of the blood between the various components of the vascular system. In this same decade of the forties, the importance of distinguishing between congestion due to heart failure and congestion occurring in the presence of a normal heart was recognized. We began also to appreciate the fact that, in many patients with heart failure, we helped the congestion but did not change the degree of heart failure.

In the 1940s too, the role of the kidney in the production of edema was appreciated and Arthur Merrill emphasized the very great changes that occur in renal blood flow and glomerular filtration in patients with congestive heart failure. He showed also that the renal blood of these patients contains an increased concentration of renin.

In the 1950s, aldosterone was recognized to be a part of the picture, but it remained for James Davis, in the early 1960s, to tie the production of aldosterone to the high concentrations of renin known to be present in the renal blood of patients with congestive heart failure. The exact weight to be put on the reduction of renal blood flow and glomerular filtration, and on endocrine and other factors in pathogenesis of the edema of heart failure, still awaits a more complete elucidation of the factors which control salt and water excretion in normal persons.

In the last few years we have begun to reevaluate the role of the lymphatics in edema. There is no evidence that the lymphatic system is diseased in congestive failure, but it may be loaded beyond its capacity. The combination of a high lymph flow produced by the disposition of the salt and water retained by the kidney in various parts of the body and a high systemic venous pressure may make a normal lymphatic system the limiting factor which determines whether edema occurs in a particular area.

The importance of arrhythmias in causing diseased heart to develop heart failure has come to the fore in this decade. Bradycardia, tachycardia and atrial fibrillation may tip the balance. New therapeutic approaches to these problems have developed. A pacemaker, driving the heart at a rate of 70 beats per minute, removed heart failure in some patients who have heart failure at a rate of 35 beats per minute. Electrical cardioversion has helped solve some of the problems of patients with atrial fibrillation. Section of aberrant connections between atrium and ventricle has solved the problem in two Duke patients with Wolff-Parkinson-White syndrome and atrial tachycardia.

The clinical teacher, knowledgeable of the pathologic physiology of heart failure and alert to therapeutic possibilities based on this knowledge, continues to attract students into his web and to give useful services to patients.[1]

•

The average patient at rest pumps about 3.3 liters of blood per minute per square meter. A person weighing around 180 pounds and six feet tall is approximately a two-meter man. His output would be about 6.5 liters per minute. The mixed A-V oxygen difference would be around four volumes of oxygen per 100cc of blood.

If this patient had chronic heart failure which would not respond to bed rest but required, in addition, sodium restriction or continuous use of mercurial diuretics, his cardiac output would be reduced at rest to around 4 liters per minute. The mixed A-V oxygen difference would rise to 6.5 liters per minute.

There is no absolute level of cardiac output below which failure is always present and above which it is never present. Whether failure is present depends on two factors: 1) whether the output of the left ventricle is high enough to keep the lungs cleaned out, and 2) whether there is enough blood pumped to normally supply all the organs.

If the patient we considered before has myxoedema, his output might fall to a level of 4 liters without evidence of heart failure. With his greatly reduced oxygen consumption, the A-V oxygen difference would remain around 4 volumes percent.

If this patient had hyperthyroidism without heart failure, his output might be 12 liters per minute with an A-V oxygen difference of 3 volumes percent. If he now developed heart failure at rest, his output will fall to 7 liters per minute with an A-V oxygen difference of 5 volumes percent. The output at rest would be enough if he had no disease but it is not enough for a patient with hyperthyroidism, and heart failure results. If one now looks at the distribution of the output one finds that in the skin flow remains high and temperature control is maintained but in other organs, particularly the kidney, the blood flow is greatly reduced.

•

There are striking similarities between congestive heart failure and hemorrhage. Hemodynamically, the only differences involve the quantity of blood in the system. Everything else is the same—arteriolar constriction, reduced cardiac output, decreased blood flow to all organs, decreased blood flow to the kidney, reduction in filtration rate, and an increase in aldosterone excretion.

. . . My guess is that the body is set up to protect itself when it is young, and it cares relatively little about the Golden Age Club. The mechanisms drawn into play when cardiac output is decreased are those which are useful when the young warrior is stabbed. Holding onto fluids and not giving up life blood when cardiac output is decreased is related to the protection of the body against hemorrhage.

. . . I guess I disagree with most people in the cardiac field, because I really believe that the hallmark of a well-treated man with vascular disease is his thinness. I, for example, am not a very obese person but I have about ·20 lb. of weight over my college weight. The reason I keep this is out of respect for my doctor. When I get heart failure, I want him to get rid of that extra 20 lb. When a patient has to live with less heart, he should live with less body.[2]

•

The clinician usually restricts the use of the term "heart failure" to those situations in which the decrease in pumping ability of the heart has lasted long enough to produce physiologic and anatomical alterations in the functions of various organs of the body. He is impressed by the fact that the heart failure may not be accompanied by any complaints which are directly referable by the patient to his heart. The patient complains of fatigue, dyspnea, edema, cough, sore liver, confusion, irregular breathing, and nocturia rather than a sore and painful heart. The fact that the failure of the heart produces such a variety of disturbances in other organs, with so little commotion in the heart, has aroused the interest of clinicians and physiologists alike.

When the heart fails, extensive adjustments occur. The clinician never concerns himself with the first changes. He is not aware of the biochemical and physical changes which occur in the heart muscle to allow it to continue to perform under the difficult conditions leading to failure. He does not detect the initial reaction to a decrease in cardiac output or the immediate consequences of the accumulation of blood in the veins. He studies the continued adjustment of the body to heart failure rather than the immediate effects of the heart failure. The physiologist is interested in the sequence of the primary events which eventually result in the clinical picture of heart failure. The clinician, never being in on the primary event, is interested in the adjustment of the body to the failure of the pump.

Physiologists and clinicians alike have been interested in the mechanisms by which heart failure leads to weight-gaining edema. In the end, it must affect the kidneys because they are the organs which are normally charged with the responsibility for excreting excess salt and water.

The patient gives us some interesting leads. He comments on the lag between drinking and voiding. He says that formerly he drank and ate during the day, that he voided the fluid he ingested during the day and that he slept at night. As failure begins, he notes that during the week when he is working he eats and drinks in the daytime but that his urine output at night has become great enough to disturb his sleep. He further notes that when he is off work from Friday afternoon to Monday morning he loses weight and is not aroused on Sunday night to void.

•

If I'm asked why the heart pumps, I have to say because it likes to. It feels more comfortable in pumping.[3]

•

We have never done much work on the problem of heart failure in acute glomerulonephritis but I will be glad to give you my own impressions from observing patients. These patients do not infrequently have heart failure. It does not seem to be the result of the hypertension per se, but it is related to the total changes occurring throughout the body as a result of the disease. The findings of an elevated venous pressure and an expanded plasma volume are not, in themselves, signs of heart failure as they may occur from the oliguria. Even pulmonary edema is not in itself a definitive sign of heart failure; that is, lesions in local capillaries can give the edema. The only way to tell whether a person with glomerulonephritis has heart failure is to determine the arterial-venous oxygen difference across the heart. If this is normal in the presence of a normal oxygen consumption, heart failure is not present, as this disease is not one of those which speeds up the circulation. If the arterial-venous oxygen difference is increased, mechanical heart failure is likely.

•

[*Hypertension*]: I saw my first patient with hypertension in the Fall of 1930. At that time the clinical association of hypertension with glomerulonephritis was appreciated. The index of my textbook of medicine (2nd edition of Cecil) listed essential hypertension and malignant hypertension.

My teachers were not certain that the increase in arterial pressure was necessarily harmful. Many doctors believed that the elevated pressure was useful in driving the blood through tissues and that if the pressure were lowered significantly, poor tissue nutrition might occur. The more thoughtful clinicians knew that the elevated pressure was not necessary for tissue perfusion. Hypertensive patients with malaria, myocardial infarction and pernicious anemia frequently became normotensive with no evidence of decreased perfusion. Today we recognize that the arteriolar narrowing which causes the increase in peripheral resistance is always reversible in all organs except the kidney. Lowering of the arterial pressure in the presence of severe renal disease may decrease the functional capacity of the kidney.

A fall in arterial pressure will occasionally cause decreased perfusion and even thrombosis when medium-sized arteries are narrowed by atheroma. Remember this is not the site of the generalized increase in peripheral resistance. The flow through the narrowed arteries decreases as the pressure head falls because in this local area ischemia has already produced local vasodilation. The surprise is not that the lowered pressure occasionally causes thrombosis. The surprise is the rarity of the event!

My next encounter with hypertension occurred during my examination for internship. Sam Levine asked me about coarctation. Fortunately for me I had read Paul White's book on the heart and was able to describe the condition. We all know how easy it is to make this diagnosis in a patient with hypertension when we think of it and how easy it is to overlook the condition when we do not feel the femoral arteries and do not take the blood pressure in the extremities.[4]

•

The abnormality in hypertension originally extends from the mitral valve in cardiac systole through the arterioles. The capillaries, veins, right heart, pulmonary vascular tree, and left atrium are not demonstrably abnormal. The first effects are mechanical, leading to cardiac hypertrophy and accelerated aging of blood vessels. Eventually, hypertension involves the capillaries and veins. The first clinical signs of capillary and venous disease are usually seen in the retina. Capillary lesions are associated with destruction of organs, particularly retina, kidneys and brain.

A given degree of arterial hypertension does not produce an equal amount of capillary disease. Lowering the blood pressure removes the mechanical strain on the heart and arteries and usually leads to capillary healing. Restriction of salt, protein, and fat, as by the rice diet, may cause the healing of capillary lesions with little effect on arterial pressure. Before organ destruction occurs, the capillary lesions are the most reversible.

When uremia and anemia enter the picture, capillary disease is accentuated.

* * * *

[*Pressures and pulses*]: The rhythmical beating of the heart and the resultant changes in flow and pressure in the arterial system have always fascinated both the lay public and physicians. Most physicians feel the pulse and record the blood pressure.

The left ventricle rhythmically forces blood into the aorta. The arterial system gains in energy with each systolic contraction. The majority of this energy is used in accelerating blood, in distending the walls of the aorta, in increasing the pressure in the arterial system and in overcoming viscous resistance to flow. The total energy added to the system cannot be calculated by the measurement of any single parameter such as lateral pressure.

The energy added to the system by ventricular contraction, which is not lost as heat, may reappear as lateral pressure. The blood can be decelerated, the aorta may decrease in volume because of elastic recoil, and the energy of pressure fed into areas of low flow may be returned to the central system to be converted into kinetic energy in areas of rapid flow.

In a closed rigid system of tubes, any increase in volume of a non-compressible liquid will cause an immediate increase in pressure throughout the system. In a distensible closed system, an increase in volume produces a bulge in the tube where the volume is increased. This bulge passes down the walls of the tubes, the lateral pressure in the tube rising in each area where the volume is increased and falling as the pressure wave moves on. Thus, in distensible tubes, an increase in volume initially causes localized rather than generalized increase in pressure. When the pressure wave reaches the end of the tube, it stops and is reflected back toward the source of origin. Eventually these oscillating waves subside and there is finally a higher, evenly distributed increase in pressure in the system.

In a collapsible system, one may make a change in pressure in the closed system either by adding fluid and increasing the volume or by compressing a portion of the system and decreasing the capacity of the system. The heart generates its pressure wave by increasing the volume of fluid in the system; a cough generates its pressure wave by decreasing the size of the aorta by external pressure.

The arterial system is made up of a system of collapsible tubes whose distensibility varies with the anatomy of the particular area examined and with the pressure within the particular segment examined. In general, the ascending and thoracic aorta increase in volume with change in pressure from diastolic to systolic levels, while the carotids, femorals and more peripheral arteries change only slightly in volume. The corollary of this is that the pressure wave travels more slowly in the aorta proximal to the renal vessels and more rapidly in the brachial and femoral vessels.

The rise in pressure along the arterial tree causes an increased rate of leak through the arterial system. The height to which the pressure wave rises in the peripheral arteries is more a function of the degree of leakiness of the system (degree of arteriolar dilatation) than it is of the elastic qualities of these vessels.

The centrally created pulse wave becomes markedly changed in form as it passes through the complex arterial system. In general, this is true of any signal which has to travel a considerable distance through different conducting media which allow different degrees of loss of power and conversion of the signal into other forms. Intuitively, one would expect the pressure wave in the aorta to be widely different from that in the dorsalis pedis artery, and accurate recording shows that the pressure waves appear much different in these two areas. [1965]

* * * *

I am familiar with the sounds you wrote me about but I don't know their origin. I assume that they are made in the artery but I have never timed them accurately enough to be certain that some are not transmitted heart sounds. The sounds are made in the neck where one can feel the carotid pulse and rule out obstruction of the common carotid artery. I do not believe that this sound eliminates the possibility of obstruction in the internal carotid artery. I see the point of your question. Can the flow in the common carotid, in the presence of disease of the internal carotid artery, vary enough in systole and diastole to produce a systolic sound? Presumably the sound, if made in a normal common carotid artery, would be caused by the increase in velocity from the contraction of the heart. Can such changes in velocity occur when one portion of the outflow tract (the internal carotid artery) is not fully patent?

Now that you have raised the question, I will be a sharper observer. We do enough arteriograms to come up with a definitive answer. [1964]

•

[*In discussing a murmur*]: You really can't say anything about how bad something is by how bad it sounds; the question is how bad it works.

* * * *

[*Fainting*]: The words *fainting* and *syncope* imply brief loss of consciousness and suggest that the fundamental disturbance must be quickly reversible. Fainting must be distinguished from more prolonged, less quickly reversible losses of consciousness. The usual cause of syncope is a sudden decrease in the blood supply to the higher nerve centers, the centers of consciousness.

Among the physiologic disturbances which may cause a decrease in the blood supply to the brain are 1) peripheral arteriolar vasodilatation; 2) failure of normal peripheral vasoconstrictor activity; 3) sharp fall in cardiac output; 4) occlusion or spasm of arteries, or temporary obstruction of carotid or other arteries to the brain; 5) decrease in blood volume.

Less frequent in the pathogenesis of true syncope are reflex effects upon the cerebral centers of consciousness. Whether these act directly on the nervous system or indirectly, by local changes in blood supply, remains to be determined.

Also less frequent in syncope (commoner in other unconscious states) but predisposing and associated factors are: changes in the constituents of the blood (chemical and metabolic causes, such as hypocapnia, hypoxia, alkalosis, acidosis, hypoglycemia, etc.)

The benign faint, produced by such stimuli as bad news, the sight of blood, hypodermic injection or venipuncture, commonly occurs while the subject is standing or sitting. The signs and symptoms of the faint result from reflex activity from a variety of sensory stimuli. The afferent impulses producing the faint may arise from the emotional content of thought or from any sensory nerve endings. Whether or not a subject faints from a given stimulus depends to a great degree upon the amount of anxiety mobilized in him by the stimulus. The intensity of the stimulus and the organ stimulated are less important.

In a few subjects a given stimulus will cause fainting no matter how often it is repeated. More commonly, the same stimulus causes less and less reaction each time. Many persons faint at the time of their first venipuncture, but never have any reaction to subsequent ones.

The clinical picture of the common faint is well known. The patient complains of a feeling of warmth in his neck and face; he becomes deathly pale and beads of sweat appear on his forehead. Yawning, belching, nausea, increased peristalsis of the gut, dilatation of the pupils, coldness of the hands and the feet and profound weakness are noted. The heart rate is usually increased. Then the arterial pressure falls rapidly. The radial pulse becomes weak and may be imperceptible, though the femoral and the carotid pulses remain full. The heart rate frequently slows dramatically. If the subject is standing he usually becomes unconscious. When the head is lowered, consciousness returns quickly. Occasionally there may be a short period of disorientation. The arterial pressure usually rises immediately when the patient is placed in the recumbent position, but at times it remains depressed for minutes or hours. Pallor, nausea, weakness and sweating frequently persist for from 30 minutes to two hours; occasionally they persist for 24 hours. If the patient stands up before recovery is complete, a precipitous fall in arterial pressure with syncope may again occur. If the subject remains upright after the loss of consciousness, clonic movements of the hands and the legs are not infrequent.

In many instances all of the phenomena usually preceding and following the loss of consciousness occur, although the patient remains conscious. To these signs and symptoms, which frequently but not necessarily terminate in syncope, the term *fainting reaction* has been applied.

The fainting reaction without loss of consciousness is frequently seen in patients who are in the horizontal position when an appropriate stimulus occurs. In the blood donor centers an occasional person loses consciousness in the recumbent position. In some of these instances convulsions with tonic and clonic phases and urinary incontinence occur in persons who never have had seizures before.

The circulatory dynamics during the fainting reaction induced in blood donors by venesection have been studied intensively during the last few years. The reaction is reflex in nature and may occur before anything is done to the donor. It may occur before the needle is inserted; after the venipuncture, but before any blood is drawn; or it may occur during or shortly after the venesection. The sharp fall in arterial pressure, the feeble radial pulse and the intense pallor suggest a sudden marked fall in cardiac output. Studies of the cardiac output by the technique of right atrial catheterization failed to confirm this. The cardiac output and the right atrial pressure did not fall as the fainting reaction occurred. The sudden fall in arterial pressure without a corresponding fall in cardiac output indicated a great decrease in peripheral resistance, as would be expected to occur with widespread arteriolar dilatation.

The demonstration that the cardiac output is well maintained in the fainting reaction accounts for the fact that the fall in arterial pressure in this condition does not usually lead to serious complications. In spite of the appearance of the patient and the low arterial pressure, the overall blood flow to the tissues remains relatively normal.[5]

•

In general, if postural hypotension is a disease of the autonomic nervous system, recovery does not occur and the patients continue to have unusual drops in blood pressure. As in most other biological phenomena, the extent to which the drop occurs and whether it produces symptoms remains variable and therefore a check on the patient's symptoms will not tell you whether his postural hypotension has disappeared.

•

A patient's complaints are generated by the reaction of his body to the stresses of living. The doctor gains useful information when, in his physical examination, he can create comparable stresses. Pathology which is not detected at rest frequently is easily demonstrated when the system is activated.

The reactivity of the autonomic nervous system, the contractility of the arterioles and veins, and the relationship between the blood volume and the capacity of the venous system can be tested by the stress of motionless standing. When the patient passes this stress test, we know that the blood volume is not seriously depleted, that the autonomic nervous system can effectively constrict both arterioles and venules, and that the smooth muscle in the arterioles and veins has the necessary vigor to contract against the pressure created by gravity. Failure to maintain a normal arterial pressure and pulse pressure against the stress of gravity is a non-specific sign of illness and requires further investigation.

Postural hypotension from volume depletion is seen in patients with bleeding and dehydration. Postural hypotension from decreased venous tone is present in many patients with acute or chronic infections. These patients with infection have normal blood volumes and good arteriolar constriction at rest, but on standing they show greater than normal fall in cardiac output. While standing, they maintain relatively normal diastolic pressure but have tachycardia and a very narrow pulse pressure. Another group of patients, those with adrenal insufficiency, may have postural hypotension from a combination of depleted plasma volume and decreased venous tone. Because of the underlying disease and the poor adjustment to gravity, patients in any of these situations—bleeding and dehydration, or acute or chronic infections, or adrenal insufficiency—are likely to have the onset of the autonomic storm that we call the common faint or vasode-pressor syncope. The heart rate slows, the arterioles in the muscles dilate and the arterial pressure falls precipitously.

Idiopathic postural hypotension results from widespread loss of function of the autonomic nervous system and produces the syndrome of postural syncope, fixed heart rate, decreased sweating and impotence. The autonomic paralysis involves the veins, the arterioles and the heart. Diabetic neuropathy may produce this syndrome in complete or incomplete form. Many drugs cause postural hypotension by varying degrees of paralysis of the autonomic nervous system. They may act at the level of the central nervous system, or at the level of the ganglia of the autonomic nervous system, or they may prevent the release of neurohumors at the nerve endings. In general, tachycardia is present in drug-induced postural hypotension.

Many patients with hypertension in recumbency have marked postural falls in arterial pressure on standing. The fall in pressure may be severe enough to cause symptoms from reduced perfusion of the brain. Therefore it is important that the standing blood pressure be known before drug therapy for hypertension is started.

Doctors can be subdivided in many ways: into listeners and talkers, into believers and non-believers, into numbers of kinds of pros and cons. Another such division might be those that take both recumbent and standing blood pressures and those that don't. I'm most impressed by those that do![6]

* * * *

[*Peripheral Vascular Disease*]: The sensations produced by ischemia to the extremity are familiar to all. When the blood supply is occluded, the part gradually becomes numb and paralyzed and we say the part has "gone to sleep". If the part is not moved, pain does not develop. The sensation at the end of the fingers becomes dulled in about 12 to 15 minutes. At that time, light pressure on the fingers may hurt, and stroking the fingertips causes an unpleasant sensation. Later, pain is dulled and, much later, analgesia develops. On release of the arterial occlusion, unpleasant tingling occurs, particularly in the fingers. This tingling is not the result of the inrush of blood into the fingers, because it occurs if blood is released only into the proximal part of the extremity. It results from changes in the main nerves of the arm during recovery. Stroking the fingers accentuates it. The paresthesias produced by the injury and recovery of the nerve from ischemia are similar to those produced by chronic disease processes involving the peripheral nerves or nerve roots.

If the extremity is exercised while the circulation is completely occluded, a continuous diffuse aching pain develops in the muscles because the sensory nerves are stimulated by the formation of stable metabolites. The pain is present during and between contractions. It is frequently described as a cramp, but the muscles are flaccid. If the contractions are continued, the muscles become tender. On release of the tourniquet, the pain disappears in a few seconds, probably as the result of the carrying away of readily diffusible metabolites.

If the brachial artery at the elbow or the femoral artery at the inguinal ligament is occluded by digital pressure for one-half hour, instead of by application of a cuff, much less change in the circulation occurs, because collateral circulation is not stopped. Loss of sensation does not occur and, on release of the occlusion, the reactive hyperemia is much less intense than with the cuff.

Embolus or thrombus in the brachial or femoral vessels frequently produces sufficient circulatory impairment to cause pain. The pain in thrombosis is indistinguishable from the pain of embolism. The pains do not occur at the site of occlusion but in the muscles and tissues distal to it. The time of onset of the pain will depend on the temperature of the part, the amount of activity, and the amount of associated vasospasm. If the part is warm and still, the limb may become numb before the muscle pain is produced. Heat applied to a limb with poor circulation may cause gangrene from 1) increased metabolism of tissue without corresponding increase in blood supply, or 2) lack of cooling effect of the blood. When heat above body temperature is applied to the skin, the blood normally acts as a cooling system; in the presence of arterial occlusion, local heating causes an immediate rise in temperature of the part.[7]

•

[*Angina Pectoris Teaches*]: The practice of medicine will always be a fascinating pursuit because of the infinite variability that occurs because the nervous system of the patient is interposed between the organs of his body and the physician who listens to the patient's complaints. Knowing that the nervous system modulates the sensory inputs and can repress, distort or amplify the signals makes the physician aware that there can be no simple relationship between complaining and disease.

Caring for patients with angina pectoris teaches the doctor a great deal of anatomy, pathology, electrophysiology, metabolism and neurophysiology which are related directly to the diseased organ. He learns also a great deal about the general organization of the nervous system and this information is useful in understanding complaints which originate in other organs than the heart.

From a general knowledge of the nervous system one would predict that there would be patients with normal hearts who would be able to pick up and amplify normal sensory inputs to a point where they would alert the conscious portion of the nervous system. The incoming stimuli might be interpreted as pain. At the other end of the spectrum we would anticipate major pathology and no complaining. The majority of patients would fall in between these two extremes.

One would predict two other types of patients. As the heart becomes scarred from disease, the nerves themselves may become ischemic and injured. One would predict that some patients who had a straightforward relationship between pain and exercise would develop much more bizarre symptoms because of sensory inputs from the diseased nerves. In these patients pain would become dissociated from the usual exercise-pain pattern and the degree of pain would no longer bear any simple relationship to the degree of coronary disease or to its rate of progression. These patients have causalgia of the heart.

In the second group, images in the nervous system do not originate from peripheral stimuli. They are formed within the nervous system and do require sensory input from the heart. The phantom limb is a case in point. This is one of the mechanisms for complaints attributed to the heart.

The careful doctor will find that this theoretical framework fits neatly with his clinical observations on patients complaining of angina pectoris. Observations on his patients with peptic ulcer, arthritis or asthma will show that in them, also, the nervous system is playing its usual tricks and that the degree of pathology will not be mirrored by the degree of the complaining.[8]

* * * *

[*The Lung*]: The lung is less protected from the environment than the skin because the lung has no "clothes". The continuous activity of the cellular elements which constantly clean up the garbage created by our environment is now well appreciated. We do not yet know enough about these cellular mechanisms to be very helpful when things go awry, but we are beginning at least to define the problem.

The location of the lungs between the systemic capillaries and the systemic arteries accounts for the importance of the lungs to the practicing physician. All organs which are diseased can come to the attention of the doctor by one of three routes. 1) The disease destroys the function of the organ in which the disease originates. 2) The primary disease invades a distal organ and causes symptoms by destroying the distant organ. 3) The primary disease causes widespread changes which are not the result of metastases. These changes may be produced by reflexes originating in the diseased organ or by biologically active materials which are carried to other organs by the blood stream. The lung is frequently destroyed by disease originating elsewhere and it is a common producer of reflexes and materials which affect other organs.[9]

REFERENCES

1. Stead EA. Medical Times **98**: 200, 1970.
2. Stead EA. Modern Medicine, Interview, August 1, 1958, p. 164.
3. Schoonmaker F, Metz E. Just Say For Me. World Press Inc., Denver, 1968.
4. Stead EA. Medical Times **94**: 766, 1966.
5. Stead EA. Chapter in Signs and Symptoms. Ed: MacBryde, J. P. Lippincott, 3rd edition, 1957, pp. 665-678.
6. Stead EA. Medical Times **95**: 1120, 1967.
7. Stead EA. Chapter in Principles of Internal Medicine. Ed: M Wintrobe. McGraw-Hill, New York, 1970, pp. 79-81.
8. Stead EA. Medical Times **98**: 201, 1970.
9. Stead EA. Medical Times **95**: 235, 1967.

• 9 •

Paid in Full by the Satisfactions of Each Day

COMMENTS ON LIVING

The past is gone, the future may never be attained. The present is real, tangible and waits to be enjoyed. In my professional life, I have never spent a year with any other purpose than to enjoy the year. If the year advanced my career, that was an additional bonus. If it did not, I had lost nothing because I had been *paid in full by the satisfactions of each day.*

•

Each person must sooner or later face up to the question, "What is the purpose of life?" The answer will have a great deal to do with the way one lives and one's relationship to others. I have never had a clear understanding of the purpose of life. I have, however, defined certain limits within which I think the answer must lie and, in this way, excluded a number of possible answers which lie outside these limits.

The purpose of life can hardly lie in the past. That period of time is over and will never recur. The purpose of life can hardly be to achieve something in the future, because the future has too little reality. In some way, the purpose of life must relate to the present. The present is real and tangible. It belongs to you; it cannot be taken away from you.

The realization that the returns from living are collected each day does modify one's behavior. One is unwilling to sacrifice everything in the present for something in the future. As a doctor, I have taken care of many parents who over many years gave everything to their children with the expectation that the children, when grown, would return this devotion in kind. In fact, as the children matured they developed their own worlds, had their own lives to live, and their own children to care for. They resented their parents' dependence on them and wished the parents had developed interests to supply pleasure from living independent of them.

Because of our belief in the present, we did not give up everything for our children. We kept some time for ourselves and always spent some part of each year away from the children. What resources we had we shared. We had our share of the free money; the children had theirs. We enjoyed our children each day and, when we put them to bed each night, the books were balanced. We had cared for them and we had enjoyed them. They owed us nothing. As the children grew older, we made it clear to them that we would support them until they were able to support themselves. After that time, we would expect to see them and their children, if all of us enjoyed the venture. When they were capable of independence, we owed them nothing and they owed us nothing. We had collected our pleasures as we went and there were no debts.

Many young men have talked with me about their plans for the next year or years. My answers have always reflected my belief in the importance of the present. If the young man is contemplating a program that he may wish he had not taken unless he achieves a particular position in some hierarchy, I advise against it. If the program pays dividends in satisfaction and pleasure while it is being pursued, he cannot lose. No matter what happens in the future, the fun of the present belongs forever to him.

I have been surprised at how rarely the young doctor, engaged in planning his career, asks the question that I judge to be of the greatest importance: "How do I plan my educational program to help me gain the greatest satisfaction out of each day of my life?" His great concern is to become technically competent, and he assumes that out of this happiness will flow. Experience shows that this may be too simple an assessment.

A doctor cannot treat diseases alone. He must care for the patient who has the disease. The doctor who wakes each morning with zest for the adventures of the day is at peace with his patients. He knows the limits which the structure of the nervous system puts on the behavior of persons. He does not expect all things from all men. He can comfortably make demands on persons capable of rising to these demands; he can comfortably make fewer demands on persons who, because of genetic background, unfavorable environment, ignorance, fear, or prejudice, have lower ceilings of performance. The doctor who enjoys the day develops a high degree of tolerance for the frailties of man and enjoys to the fullest the triumph of individuals. The course of education selected by the young doctor should be one which teaches him to enjoy the people who have the illnesses he has learned to treat. This is the only way to assure that the work of each day will bring true satisfaction.

To keep one's perspective on the problems of living, one needs to have some sense of the geological time scale. The most famous men of recorded history occupy very few moments in our thoughts. How few of us spend any time thinking about Alexander the Great or Julius Caesar! Within a few million years, all traces of them could disappear from the thoughts of any living man. The purpose of life can hardly be to obtain fame, because it is too impermanent. Events which add to the enjoyment of the day may bring distinction and fame. The achievement of fame and distinction at the expense of the enjoyment of the day does not bring happiness.

The knowledge of the uncertainty of the future does influence the direction of one's life. A doctor knows that he or anyone else may die before a new day dawns. The wise man is not disturbed by this. He does each day what he wants to do and, if the date of his death were known to him, he would not need to change his plans. He has planned his life with the knowledge of its impermanence. If he lives in the present, he need have no fear of the future.

A doctor's philosophy does have an effect on his practice. I believe that young people can be "insurance poor" and give up too much of the present in caring about the future. I am not enthusiastic about burdening my patients with too many *don'ts* when I have no way of knowing what will remove them from this earth. All preventive measures are wasted when the patient dies from another cause before the diseases which were being prevented would have actually interfered with his way of life.

Many persons will come to doctors complaining of certain ailments. The doctor often does not find, in any of his testing, disturbances in function great enough to account for the complaining. He will frequently find asymptomatic diseases which may at some future time cause symptoms. Obesity, hypertension, abnormal blood lipids, elevated uric acid, and an abnormal glucose tolerance test are common findings. In his search for a solution to the complaints of the patient, the doctor may institute a regimen of preventive medicine in a person who sought medical help in the first place because he was barely able to keep his nose above water. The preventive measures cost money, require energy from the patient, and in no way relieve the situation which drove him to the doctor. A doctor with an eye to the present would never initiate programs aimed at the future until the patient was back on an even keel.

I have had little enthusiasm for the annual physical examination which is strongly test and x-ray oriented. It is a kind of negative medicine which puts me to sleep. On the other hand, I am keenly aware that our bodies are undergoing continual change, and that our behavior and our interaction with our environment change with the years. It is worthwhile for one to have an evaluation of his body and how he is using it to determine whether he is getting as much as possible out of each day's living.

Department heads should work harder to devise social systems that recognize certain biologic facts. They do not appreciate fully that all manifestations of behavior are a function of the structure of the nervous system. The structure is a mixture of nonreversible and reversible units. The number of reversible units decreases with age. Every five years, enough change occurs in each of us that, from the viewpoint of body-environment interaction, we can be considered to be a new person. This new person will have different perspectives, different aptitudes, a different interaction with the environment. The returns from the day will decrease unless we are allowed to change our activities as our bodies change. No one knows the direction or the magnitude of the changes that will occur in a young faculty member as he grows older. All we know is that change will occur, and we should structure our affairs to profit by the change. Many times the social structure is so tight that only penalties accrue as change occurs. A young man starting his career may be able to offer many contributions before he retires. He may begin as an excellent teacher of beginning students and in time he may evolve into an excellent bioscientist. Later, clinical interest becomes stronger and he becomes an increasingly important clinician; he now gives up a large part of his laboratory space to a younger person and takes a more prominent role in advanced graduate training. In due time he becomes an outstanding leader in his area of clinical specialization and devotes more time to national affairs. This type of evolution requires a flexible system of funding so that the man can be supported from different sources as his functions change. In time, the teaching and research dollars are replaced by patient care and administrative dollars.

Each intern, resident, or fellow has some particular environment with which he can interact best. The head of a large educational program has the responsibility for identifying this circumstance. He must guide the young men to recognize their potentialities and limitations so that they can live comfortably with these realities. False notions that one kind of work is more honorable than another must be stripped away. Young men must be persuaded to determine the personal satisfactions—the returns of each day—which will come from a variety of different careers. Each career, however different, may be equally honorable. The returns to different persons in satisfaction may be widely different. The career which has been completely satisfying to the mentor may be a disaster for his pupil. An instructor interested in the joy of the present will not try to mold in his own image the young men whom he encounters.[1]

* * * *

I think we're becoming slowly more aware of the fact that the fetus is part of the mother while they're sitting there together.

•

With us always has been the question of when the life of the individual begins and when society begins to protect this life because it has gained the dignity of a human being. Eggs and sperm die separately without any pangs of conscience.[2]

•

The receptivity of the nervous system is a wonderful thing. Having a young boy, seeing him run around all day, and then seeing him under the covers at night makes this obvious to me.[3]

•

Children are going to have to be content with less than their parents have; they already have less land.

•

Low income housing means low income people. The only way to stop it is to not build the houses.

•

Increasing population increases the locked doors. This is society's way of placing more restrictions on the population.[3]

•

We cause most of the things that happen to us.

•

Repetitious behavior must lead to satisfaction or it wouldn't be done.

•

That man is not a farsighted biological creature is evidenced by the way he kills off all the able in war.[3]

•

The right to fail is a great right. I always like to fail in a way that I'd be smarter. That way I won't fail the same way again. Clearly it's more fun to succeed that to fail.

•

Emotional debts are much harder to collect than other debts.

•

People get mixed up on whether it was bad or whether it was hard.[3]

•

There are two fallacies I know that lead people to thinking they're better than others. One, people who are successful believe they did it. And people feel that physical structure puts a limitation on performance and this makes people feel they're worthy and others are unworthy.

•

The only people who don't have serious family problems are those you don't know.

•

The man who must know every fact, who is destroyed if he must admit ignorance, is at the mercy of everyone who asks him a question.

•

Biological systems are not changed by the academic rank, harsh words or the most recent article read.[3]

•

One of the men on our staff decided many years ago that a certain post in the hospital was in the wrong place. I would have to agree with him that the post is in the wrong place but, unlike the other man, I've found it just as easy to walk around it, and he still bumps into it every day.[3]

•

If one finds that he is having difficulty with the people around him, then he must be having difficulty as a man. There are many people who are problem creators.[3]

•

One of the interesting things about going through the day is that you personalize everybody else's actions and think his interaction is toward you, when really they themselves are just trying to get through the day and everything is impersonal, with interactions with others being just incidental.

•

The best way to get a difficult job done is face to face or ear to ear. Sending notes is never satisfactory.[3]

•

What determines how tired we are is not usually the amount of physical work but how many times we interact with others, how much time we spend trying to get someone to do something and him trying to get us to do something.

•

Person to person interface is where most energy is spent.

•

Traditionally, people have good thoughts before they become old, or never any . . .

•

I have always thought the last part of education is always more fun than the first, and you like it better when you're older.

•

If you find today dull, you'll find tomorrow dull.

•

The ability to deny the worst that's going to happen to you is what keeps you going over the years.

•

I think, if you think back on how to be profound in a situation, you can be only as human as you actually are. You can't think thoughts you haven't thought before, or be a different person than you've been before. There's no magic to any given moment.

•

As you die, I know nothing to do except to die as you have lived.

•

Dying is not terribly hard to do; everybody is capable of passing the course. However, you want as few scars as possible left with the living.

•

There is a cost to dying. The longer you live the higher the cost.

•

Death is not to be reckoned with in the last hours of life, but all through life. One cannot look directly at the sun or at death.[3]

•

Any one of us may die on the way to staff conference. Get the most satisfaction you can get from each of the moments you are here.

* * * *

It is interesting to see how cultural patterns develop. I have great trouble in moving people out of New York City to our area, but those who do move become equally difficult about moving back. . .

•

What's culture in North Carolina is insanity in New York.[3]

•

When I was young, I never imagined then that anyone would ever pay me such a good salary for doing exactly what I wanted to do.[3]

•

I don't honestly think that I can call what I do work.

•

If you're doing what you want to do, you're never tired.

•

I'm not so immune to the simple pleasures of life that I don't enjoy hearing a young man say that he has learned a lot from me but, realistically, I know it's not so. Bright men teach themselves.[3]

•

I have no quarrel with the notion of father figures. I've been one myself for years.[3]

•

The world is made up of believers and non-believers. For now I'll be a non-believer.

•

Nearly always I start out about as skeptical as I can.

•

I have more fun talking than you have listening.

•

A good clinician ceases to make a distinction between work and play. A child equates play with good and work with bad. When a physician does this, clinical medicine becomes intolerable for him.[3]

•

The doctor must mold himself to a great variety of people.

•

No greater opportunity, responsibility or obligation can fall to the lot of a human being than to become a physician. In the care of the suffering, he needs technical skill, scientific knowledge and human understanding. He who uses these with courage, with humility and with wisdom will provide a unique service for his fellow man and will build an enduring edifice of character within himself. The physician should ask of his destiny no more than this; he should be content with no less.[3]

•

Clinical medicine is a demanding mistress; when a physician becomes intolerant of the demands made on him, the affair is short-lived.[3]

* * * *

The way to get things done around here is to tell Bess.

REFERENCES

1. Stead EA. Chapter in Hippocrates Revisited. Ed: RJ Bulger, Medcom Press, 1973, New York, pp. 126-129.
2. Stead EA. Medical Times **95**: 1173, 1967.
3. Schoonmaker F, Metz E. Just Say For Me. World Press Inc., Denver, 1968.

PART II
Biography

Each Year I Cheerfully Send Emory A Check

BIOGRAPHICAL NOTES

I have always been grateful for Emory, my alma mater. This small, struggling college had the audacity to attach to itself a failing proprietary medical school. At the time I entered, it was on and off the probation list. It was 1928 and the Great Depression had already begun in the South. The only question anyone asked when I applied for admission was, "Son, can you borrow the money for tuition?" I said that the Atlanta Rotary Club would lend me the money. *Each year I cheerfully send Emory a check.* No Emory medical school, no Dr. Eugene Stead.

•

In my family we grew up thinking that if you wanted to get up in the morning and do something nobody could stop you.

•

The only times I ever won prizes was at the YMCA. I had the biggest ears and I could put on my shoes and socks faster than anyone else.

•

I studied in high school because I found learning fun. In college I took biology because my sister's boyfriend pointed out that one particular assistantship was the best-paying undergraduate job on the campus. I was appointed to that position at the end of my first year in college.

I entered medicine because it offered more intellectual challenge than any other area on my college campus. I lived seven years in a white suit and had a wonderful time. I gave the best care to my patients that I could, because I enjoyed doing it. I suggested to my young colleagues that they try my way of doing things because they might discover that excellent performance has its own reward. I do not remember suggesting to anyone that they do anything for humanity.

I learned that, just as many people like to fish or play golf, I like to work with my head.

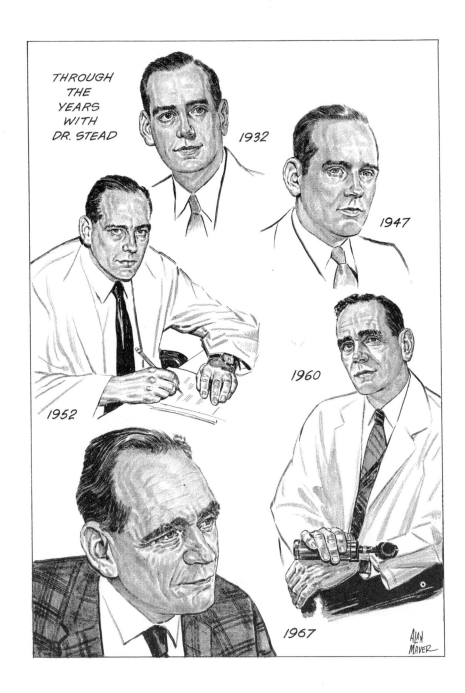

THROUGH THE YEARS WITH DR. STEAD

1932

1947

1952

1960

1967

ALAN MAVER

* * * *

M.D., 1932, Emory   *James Paullin*

My first professor of Medicine was also our family doctor. He first showed me in his work that the family doctor of the future was going to be the intelligent, interested internist. He made home calls rarely, but he knew every member of my family, and no medical attention was ever sought without first reviewing the problem with him. Every Tuesday and Wednesday morning he was at Grady Hospital. His patients respected his desire for continued growth as a doctor and never begrudged him this time. He was interested in medical politics and repeatedly demonstrated that all human group endeavor involves some type of political activity. He was a medical politician in the best sense of the word and all of American medicine profited by his broad interests.[1]

•

In his study of symptomatology, my first chief appreciated the complexity of medicine in modern society. He was aware of the frequency with which multiple factors operate to produce disease and symptoms. He became interested in the mechanisms by which emotional reactions cause the patient to feel abnormal.

* * * *

1932–34, Medicine, Brigham   *Henry Christian*

Under the guidance of my second chief, the Peter Bent Brigham medical resident staff developed many leaders in medicine. The atmosphere of the Brigham was one that gave honor to scholarship.

He was successful in the development of leaders because he fostered in his residents a willingness to take the initiative. His attitude was not that the Brigham service was good because of the senior staff, but that it was good in spite of the senior staff. He relied heavily on the fact that he had pulled into his net many bright boys from all sections of the country, and he expected them to produce. I have never seen men more conscious of their ability to learn for themselves than those resident groups assembled by him.

•

Early in my internship I was walking down the Brigham pike with Dr. Sam Levine when Dr. Joe Aub stopped him to ask him to see a young woman with fever of unknown etiology. He wanted to know whether the patient had bacterial endocarditis. Dr. Levine listened very carefully to her heart, determined that she had no murmur, and told Dr. Aub he did not have to worry about subacute bacterial endocarditis. Within a few days

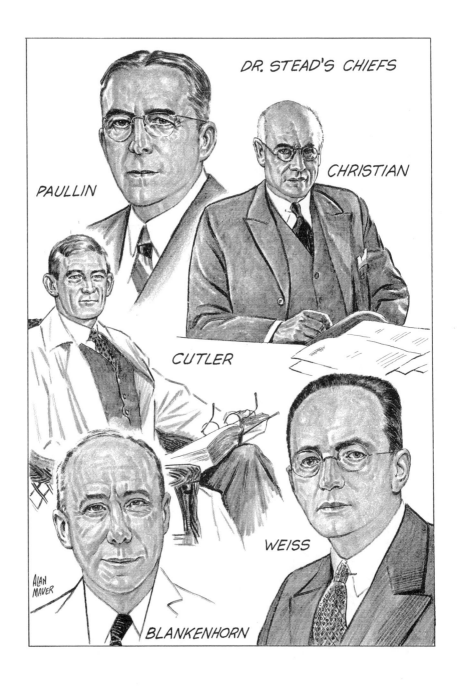

DR. STEAD'S CHIEFS

PAULLIN

CHRISTIAN

CUTLER

WEISS

BLANKENHORN

ALAN
MAVER

a pleural effusion developed and in time the diagnosis of tuberculosis was established. This old rule: *no murmur, no subacute*, is still useful. It may fail when the infected endothelium is not in the heart as in a peripheral A-V fistula, in patients with endothelium damaged by myocardial infarction, and in some elderly patients.[2]

* * * *

1934–35, Surgery, Brigham   *Elliot Cutler*

My third chief, under whom I served a 16-month surgical internship, was loved and honored by all of his staff, even the lowly intern. On his service I discovered how hard surgeons work, and I learned that those long hours in the operating room use up the time which the internist loves to spend talking with his patients and teaching.[1]

* * * *

1935–37, Medicine, Cincinnati General Hospital   *Marion Blankenhorn*

My fourth chief gave to me my basic interest in clinical observation. Under his guidance, the history and physical examination came alive. His teaching centered around the patient and he destroyed once and for all my interest in dry clinics. He gave his resident a very free hand in running the service, and from him I learned not only to do my own work but how to get other people to work.[1]

•

[*Letter from EAS to Dr. Blankenhorn, 1955*]:   What a flood of memories comes to me as I begin this letter! I came to your service as an immature uncertain assistant resident and I left it 18 months later as a confident doctor. The sense of being at home in medicine which grew into me on your service has lasted throughout the years.

I remember many small things that you have long since forgotten: the man with the chronic emphysema and contracted chest who I thought had atelectasis from bronchial obstruction: you asked for a needle and out came the pus; the first sympathectomy in a desperately ill patient with hypertension; the patient apparently recovering from pneumococcal pneumonia in whom you heard the early diastolic whiff indicating the development of bacterial endocarditis.

I have never forgotten the support that you gave to your resident. He was free to run the service and to try out his own ideas. For me it was a year of great growth in my relationship to other people. For the first time, I began to understand how to work with other people and to get them to help me.

Your service has grown greatly since my time as resident. Your staff, your residents and your students have spread the tales of your skill far and wide. Even many of your mannerisms are affectionately imitated the country over.

We regret that the time for formal retirement is approaching, but we know that you will keep your hands in many things.

•

I was chief resident at Cincinnati General when Soma Weiss came to visit with us five days. I saw many patients with Soma and had the opportunity to know him personally. I had planned to go to Atlanta to practice. When Soma left he suggested that I come instead to the Thorndike as his research fellow. I told him I'd like to but I had certain debts to pay off and that I had to have an income of $1800. He said no fellow had ever been paid $1800. I said, "Don't worry about it; I don't have anyone else I want to work for. If you find another $900, let me know." (He was willing to pay me $900.) In April I got a wire, "Found $900." I wired back "See you in July." And that's how I got to the Thorndike.

* * * *

1937–39, Boston City
1939–41, Brigham   *Soma Weiss*

My fifth and last chief was Soma Weiss. By that time the clay was better worked and more ready for the molding, and Soma taught me many things.

From Soma I learned the importance of keeping down artificial barriers which interfere with learning. Whoever knew the most about the problem—second-year student, instructor or visitor—was cock of the walk for the moment. Soma achieved remarkable give-and-take with everyone contributing to the learning pot and everyone taking knowledge back out.

Soma never forgot that the function of a university service was to train men and the output of research was always secondary to this main objective. He carried on research with the resident staff for its effect on their thinking. Research with the older staff was a means of keeping their minds alert and their teaching interesting.[1]

•

[*Letter to William B. Castle, 1957*]: Your appointment as the Minot Professor of Medicine and the occasion of your sixtieth birthday makes me review the many happy memories of my Thorndike days. I wrote my first paper in June after coming to work with Soma the preceding September. As Soma was away, the job of helping me editorially fell to you with an able assist from Miss Shorley. The experience was a delightful one for me. Without knowing the technical details, you grasped immediately what was being done and why, and I profited as much by your comments on how to write up the material as I did from doing the work.

I point out to my students that I learned two particular things of great value from you. The first was not to be too compulsive about knowing everything. The second was how to conduct an exercise in thinking without knowing everything about the problem. I can still see you approaching a clinical problem and dividing it into the areas known and understood by you and the group of students and house staff; the areas probably known by others with knowledge available from proper use of the library; and the areas probably not known by anyone but areas which could be approached experimentally.

•

When I went to the Thorndike in 1937, I wanted $200 to build a foot plethysmograph. I filled out an application and Soma took it to Henry Christian, who approved the application from the Milford Fund which was under his control. I opened the laboratory at the Brigham in 1939, with two rooms, several mercury sphygmomanometers, several syringes and needles, a homemade hand-operated title table and a Klett colorimeter. Life was both simple and interesting.

Soma had a genuine and sustained interest in the persons who worked with him as well as in the work they accomplished. It's difficult to say whether he was a hard taskmaster. He worked a long day and enjoyed it. The students, house staff and research fellows worked long days and nights and enjoyed it.

Soma demonstrated the importance of the undergraduate student in our own learning. Repeated efforts to explain to the student the basic mechanisms of health and disease kept before us the extent of our own ignorance and made us examine critically the premises on which we based our glibly quoted clinical aphorisms. We learned the importance of appreciating what is not known about a condition as well as what is known.

This same use of teaching as a learning device was employed with the resident staff. Every intern and resident taught students, not because there was no other way to teach the student but because of the learning value to the resident group.

In the laboratory, Soma taught us the value of not giving up too easily and yet he kept us from beating our heads against a stone wall on a problem for which methods then known were inadequate.

•

Soma maintained a great interest in the symptoms which patients present. He realized that the learning of medicine from the practice of medicine was dependent entirely upon an accurate evaluation of the cause of the patient's complaint. A patient with heart disease who complains of shortness of breath may have congested lungs which are causing the dyspnea, or he may be short of breath from anxiety, or he may have independent lung disease. If the doctor mistakes emotional dyspnea for congestive failure, he learns nothing from treating the patient.

Soma not only knew what he wanted to do, but he knew how to get it done. He didn't rail at the political moves necessary to keep the city fathers happy. He knew that all the ruling powers were people and he enjoyed handling people. It made little difference whether they were sick folk or people with power who needed education. He showed that administration was a necessary function and could be fun in its own way.[1]

•

[*Letter to James V. Warren, 1977*]:   What a great adventure life has been! The Thorndike years under Soma Weiss were important to us all. I well remember the tall, attractive young student waiting for his internship to begin who, along with Lew Dexter and Soma, initiated us into the mysteries of toxemia. That excursion into the vagaries of obstetrics resulted in the collaborative efforts between the Brigham and the Lying In Hospital which are still active.

The Brigham years were equally important. When Dick Ebert and Jim Warren joined hands with me, my investigative career really began.

•

We live in a different world from 1937–41 when Soma Weiss was at his peak. Soma's principal disciples were few in number because funding was difficult and appointments few.

Myron Prinzmetal from the West Coast; Bill Bean who is now in Galveston; Robert Wilkins, professor of medicine at Boston University; Richard Ebert, professor of medicine at University of Minnesota; Dick Capp in practice in Chicago; Paul Kunkel in practice in Connecticut; Jim Warren at Ohio State; Lewis Dexter at the Peter Bent Brigham; and Ted Astwood who is now in practice in Bermuda are the persons I know who actually worked in the laboratories which were at Soma's disposal. Jack Myers and Paul Beeson were chief residents under Soma.

Soma was head of the 2nd medical service at the Boston City Hospital and had teaching contact with house officers there between 1929 and 1939. He had Tuesday night rounds which covered every medical and neurological ward at the City, and young people from all the Boston hospitals and from all the medical schools in Boston attended them.

Jack Gibson, who remained at the Brigham as a research associate, Charles Janeway, professor of pediatrics at the Boston Children's Hospital, John Romano, professor of psychiatry, and I moved to the Brigham when Soma took over as the Hersey Professor.

Tinsley Harrison and Soma Weiss were well-trained doctors who were interested in the symptoms produced by disease processes. They knew that all symptoms were, by definition, intertwined with the nervous system. They rapidly discovered that the circulatory system was tied in closely with the nervous system and that there were many reflexes which were disturbed in disease. They brought physiology to the bedside, and they were fascinating teachers who contrasted brilliantly with the persons trained primarily in classification of disease and routine memorization of signs and symptoms. Their impact on students and house staff was tremendous. They were movers of men rather than great scientists in their own right.

The ability to read German easily and fluently gave Soma a real advantage over most of his colleagues. He kept abreast of the European literature. The work of Heyman on the carotid sinus intrigued him, and he was searching for clinical application of this knowledge long before most Americans were aware of baroreceptors and chemoreceptors.

Soma had a genuine and sustained interest in the persons who worked with him as well as in the work that they accomplished.

•

Hyperplasia, adenoma or carcinoma of islet cells may cause hypoglycemia with delirium and coma. The first patient I saw with an islet cell adenoma was under treatment for an illness supposedly related to environmental stress. His wife complained that he drove the car recklessly and that later he could not remember having done so. He was an anatomy diener and in time was found sleeping in the vats with the cadavers. This behavior, alternating with periods of entirely normal behavior, led to more careful history taking. It was quickly established that food prevented the delirium and starvation produced it. The laboratory data were confirmatory. John Romano, now professor of psychiatry at the University of Rochester, and I studied the behavior of this gentleman during starvation. We exercised him periodically on a bicycle and some time during the night precipitated a hypoglycemic attack. The following Saturday Romano presented him at grand rounds to Soma Weiss and Walter Cannon, the distinguished professor of physiology at Harvard. I had drawn a chart showing the amount of work we had used to intensify the hypoglycemia. Unfortunately I shifted the decimal point and the amount of work recorded on the chart was hardly enough to have a physiologic effect. To Romano's great relief Cannon made no comment, but John has never let me forget the episode. Our gentleman had a name that rhymed with eaten. Romano's summary of this somewhat protracted study was: ". . . should have eaten!"[3]

•

There are several possible mechanisms [for heart failure], and each has its proponents. The mechanism was first thought to be simple failure behind the right ventricle. With heart failure, the blood begins to accumulate first behind the left ventricle and then, as heart failure continues to develop, behind the right ventricle. As a result, it was suggested, there is a rise in venous pressure causing fluid to be pushed out into the tissues, thus producing edema. Essentially, the thesis is that the blood stream becomes depleted of water because of high venous pressure and the water is not available to the kidney for excretion. Richard Ebert and I investigated this type of heart failure while at Peter Bent Brigham Hospital in Boston. We tried to make our own heart failure by leaning up against a wall to increase venous pressure and drinking salt water. We alternated on the wall, made a lot of measurements, but we never produced heart failure. We could never get the increase in blood volume. We eventually produced edema, but we never increased the blood volume.[4]

•

I well remember the first patient we treated successfully with penicillin. The clinical diagnosis was obvious, the organism was strep viridans, and Paul Beeson was freshly armed with penicillin. The patient had unequivocal heart failure. Paul, with his usual wisdom, was concerned about the heart failure. I cockily assured him that all he had to do was make the heart valves sterile and I would take care of the heart failure. He did his part but, in spite of my best efforts, the patient died of heart failure. Patients with heart failure at the time treatment is started still have a very bad prognosis.[2]

•

As do so many of us, I remember with pleasure the intellectual stimulus that I received at the Thorndike. The students on the 2nd and 4th services had a great experience and one which was not duplicated on the other medical services available to the Harvard students. The control of the clinical research unit and of the clinical service allowed the Thorndike unit to develop its own philosophy.

If the Thorndike of old could rise we would all cheer. It may be that it is impossible to recreate the past and we will have to be satisfied with our memories.

* * * *

1942–47, Emory

The year 1942 opened with me facing up to the fact that I was going to Emory with a total budget of $23,500 and very little chance of succeeding in academic medicine. I was very hesitant about asking people to come to Emory. The turning point in my career came one night when Jim Warren, Eddie Miller, John Hickam and Abner Golden announced that they would

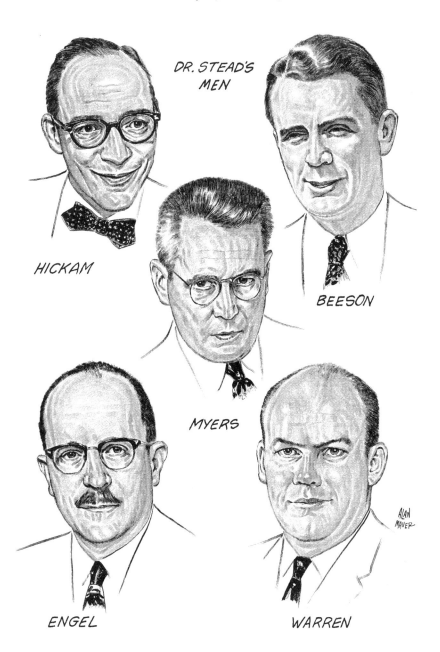

DR. STEAD'S
MEN

HICKAM

BEESON

MYERS

ENGEL

WARREN

be in Atlanta in July. I said that I doubted the wisdom of that decision. I was informed that I was not being asked for my opinion: I was merely being informed about what would happen.

The Grady days were glorious days. We were very short of money. We had to have a defense contract to study shock in order to survive. Al Blalock visited us and recommended that we be given a small contract to study shock in animals and that we try to develop a program to study shock in man. Jim Warren suggested that he visit Cournand and see if the cardiac catheter was the tool we needed to develop a program to study shock at the Gradys.

After Jim's visit of several weeks with Cournand, we were able to propose a program to the War Resources Development Board for the study of shock in patients. Our first budget grossly underestimated our costs. We were saved by a transcription error. A decimal point was shifted one point to the right and we had just enough money for the project. This project allowed the air conditioning of the basement laboratories and we at least were protected from heat and from the dust of the cars parked in the dirt lot between our basement laboratories and Coca Cola Place.

I can still feel the excitement of the ventures of the team of Warren, Merrill, Brannon, Weens and Stead. The decision to study patients with heart failure was always with us. Looking back over those times I can think of only one major opportunity that we dropped. We did not link the increased renin output of patients with chronic heart failure with the control of aldosterone.

•

[*Re pericardial tamponade*]: I used to live in the icepick world down in Grady Hospital. We always tapped them before sending them to operation because sometimes the hole would be small enough and the problem would not recur.

•

At Emory our first assignment was to arrange the department's teaching program within the block of time allotted to the department of medicine. We decided first to free the faculty of any compulsion to cover a very large block of knowledge. We would teach from the patients and attach knowledge already acquired to the particular patient the student was caring for. The student would re-investigate those phases of the basic sciences which applied to the particular patient and learn that part of clinical medicine which applied to the same patient. The patient would be the stimulus for learning, because this stimulus would last as long as the student practiced medicine. The role of the faculty would be to see that the student enjoyed his learning experiences and developed a desire to continue them. This system of "slow" learning required that the faculty be willing to tolerate ignorance of many specific areas of medicine. If we laid down no hard and fast body of knowledge that had to be learned, we could not criticize the student for ignorance of a particular fact. We had to base our judgments on his ability to use those facts we did have. If he could manipulate these facts, tear them down and rebuild new structures with them—in short, think—we would be satisfied.

My Emory students are now well established in practice, teaching and research. I have heard from them often about their experiences as interns in other hospitals. They realized that they had memorized fewer facts than students from many other schools; but they were not dismayed when new situations arose and they were satisfied with their ability to learn from each new experience. I am satisfied that their performance since graduation vindicates the method by which they were taught.

Thus my Emory years were spent in freeing the members of the department from the need for compulsive coverage of the field of internal medicine and in freeing the medical student from the idea that he worked because he was in school. Instead, the student learned to work for the fun of learning and to give his patients good care.

The use of research as an important component of education can be defended only anecdotally. I went to Grady to a house staff who had had access to the library. They were very widely read. Their reading was totally uncritical. Never having had a hand in creation of knowledge, they were not aware of the pits into which all authors at one time or another fall. They believed everything they read and were puzzled by the fact that one paper said one thing and a second just the opposite. I decided at that time not to engage in major educational ventures without a faculty engaged in creating new knowledge and publishing it in well-edited journals.

•

When I went to Grady Hospital, the heads of the colored and white hospitals said there wasn't a place for me. So I got up a little earlier and went to bed a little later and before long I ran Grady. The world belongs to those who work a little harder.

* * * *

1947–67, Duke
   Expenses of Dr. Eugene Stead, Jr. to Durham, North Carolina
      June 30, 1947
         Plane fare, Atlanta to Raleigh-Durham $19.15
         Miscellaneous expenses   5.31
                                              ———————
                                                  $24.46

•

In January 1947 I came to Duke Medical School as professor of medicine, chairman of the Department of Medicine, and physician-in-chief of Duke Hospital. I was directly responsible for the care of staff patients and for any private patients who came to me for medical services. The medical students, interns, and residents supervised the care of the staff patients under guidance from the senior staff and me. They also helped with the care of private patients, both those of my own and of other members of the staff. From the beginning, the students and house staff pointed out to me that edematous patients and patients with malignant hypertension treated by Kempner with his rice diet did better than the patients treated by me with digitalis, diuretics and moderate sodium restriction. My own observations supported theirs and, with the aid of the Durham-Orange County Heart Association, Bernard C. Holland and I opened a Heart House to provide rice diet therapy for the staff patients of Duke Hospital. We made no new advances. We did have the satisfaction of seeing many of our previously difficult patients do remarkably well.[5]

•

The Duke University medical school is Dr. Davison's school. He was there before the buildings were built, before the books were bought for the library, before an administrative staff was assembled, and before a single faculty appointment was considered. On all of our walls under the paint, one finds inscribed, "Davison was here".

Under Dr. Davison's guidance the medical school grew into a community of scholars concerned with all phases of knowledge. He concerned himself with the practice of medicine in the state, the South, and the nation. He built an outstanding library. He operated a clinical center which has steadily grown until it has a worldwide reputation. He developed a system of private university clinics which bring a steady flow of visitors to Duke to study their operation. He spread pediatricians far and wide over the land and laid the basis for the development of a children's clinical center at Duke. He recognized the vitalizing impact of research upon the corporate body of the medical school, but properly pointed to its inordinate demands. There were no slaves or masters on his form sheet.

Dr. Davison had the ability to delegate responsibility to others. He required a high level of performance, demanding of others the same standards of excellence which he had for himself. Under his guidance the school was not paternalistic. If a faculty member failed at Duke, the credit for the failure belonged to him and not to the dean. If a faculty member succeeded at Duke, the dean made it clear that the credit for the success belonged to the faculty member and not to the dean.

Dr. Davison separated his personal feelings from his responsibilities to the school. He did not hesitate to state his own adverse opinion of an individual. If his performance in the school was good, he supported him while disliking him. He was interested in assembling an outstanding faculty rather than a social club.

Dr. Davison operated informally. He was known to the faculty simply as "Dave". He did not depend on props for dignity. Coatless and tieless, he was always the Duke medical school. He believed that no rules should ever be written down if it were possible to avoid doing so. Why limit the future by the vision of the past?

Dave always knew that good administration required a personal touch. Accomplishments of faculty members, wives or children were acknowledged by a note from the dean. Every patient with any interest in Duke was visited by him. In truth, the man seemed to have eyes in the back of his head, and ears everywhere.

As with all good administrators, his word was his bond. He carried a little notebook attached to his wallet. Once he agreed to a course, it was noted in the book. The matter was then as good as accomplished.[6]

* * * *

When I came to Duke in January 1947, I inherited a vigorous clinical faculty. With the exception of the neurologists and one cardiologist, I could not have selected a better clinical staff. The tradition at Duke was that the clinical departments would have no laboratories and that all laboratory research would be done in collaboration with the basic science departments. This tradition was being broken by the development of laboratories by Beard and Grimson in Surgery and by Nicholson and Kempner in Medicine. Beard was supported by research funds that he created and by funds from the Department of Surgery. Nicholson, Kempner and Grimson created the majority of their funds in practice.

With the exception of the chairman, all members of the Department of Medicine were paid either $3,000 per year (Ruffin and Hansen-Pruss) or $2,500 per year. They created the rest of their income from practice and contributed a portion of this income to the building fund, which was spent over the signature of the clinical chairmen, and to the departmental fund which was spent over my signature. There were no persons except the chairman who were paid enough money to allow them to have uninterrupted time for research. Each member of the department met his assigned teaching duties willingly and easily. Any variation in these assignments was difficult to meet without a month's notice because of patient appointments.

The faculty did not use the private patients for teaching. This seemed inefficient to me. Granted that the doctor teaching and caring for his private patient would use more time per patient than he did if he were only caring for the patient, there would be a net gain over the time lost if he cared for the private patient and then taught on a ward patient. The moving of more teaching activity to the private arena would make more room for new faculty members who would be paid on a fixed salary. They would engage in practice on a fixed time basis and not increase their income if they increased their time in practice beyond the agreed-upon limit. This would allow the development of research laboratories in the Department of Medicine and allow me to have greater flexibility in assigning duties to the staff.

Traditionally the Department had used the money contributed to the departmental fund for a series of further benefits, ranging from the support of research assistants and secretaries to travel. The idea that the fund be used for the full-time support of new faculty members less dependent on funds created by each new faculty member was not in their thinking.

My problem then was to enlarge the physical plant and the teaching and research activities of the Department without interfering with the growth of our excellent clinical staff. Looking over the financial picture I was impressed that a group of highly competent clinicians were receiving an income greatly in excess of anyone in the rest of the University or in the basic science areas of the medical school. It was easily determined that the small amount of money paid to these clinicians could be recovered by simply improving their working conditions by air-conditioning the medical private diagnostic clinic. I could divert the $45,000 to be saved into income for my new faculty less committed to medical practice. The salaries of this new faculty would be in line with the basic science faculty. I thought that the $45,000 at issue would be better defended against a predatory medical dean or University president under these new arrangements. I made the recommendations for the shift in money to Dr. Davison. He said that this was unacceptable to the clinical faculty. It hit me at a time when I was irritable and restless. I submitted my resignation, feeling that there was too much bickering about a small amount of money.

I had not appreciated that the clinical staff in spite of their favorable income situation had always resented the fact that Dave raised money for the preclinical staff and not for them. The removal of the $2,500 to $3,000 stipend meant to them that they were being made less important to the medical school and University. This thought had never penetrated into my thinking. I was trying to protect the money so that the charges against patient income would not have to be increased.

Time has proved me wrong. No predatory dean or University president

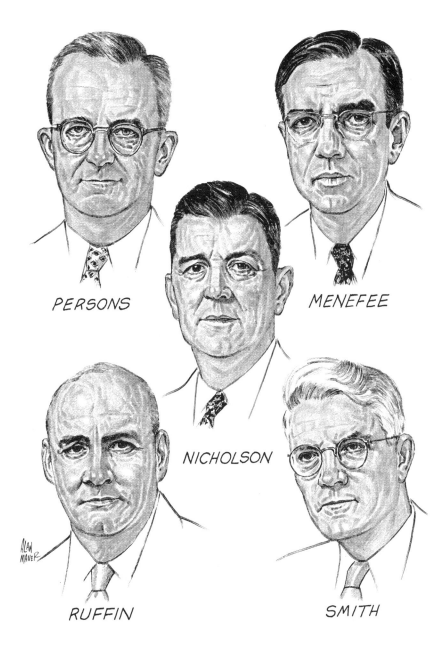

PERSONS

MENEFEE

NICHOLSON

RUFFIN

SMITH

Senior Staff, Duke Department of Medicine, 1947

has ever attacked those small stipends. I would have been correct in 95 out of 100 schools. I was wrong at Duke.

Two days after my resignation, Wiley Forbus came by to teach me a few of the facts of life. He reviewed the opportunities that lay in front of me at Duke. He recounted the times he had made errors in judgment and had had to back down. He showed me that in the end these episodes had been beneficial to him and had facilitated his growth as a person. He urged me to withdraw my resignation. I did so in a letter to Dave. He replied that he had no power to allow me to withdraw the resignation. The Executive Committee would have to vote to accept the resignation or to decline to accept it.

The matter was put on the agenda of the next Executive Committee meeting. Dave was not yet ready for the vote and he managed to have an Executive Committee meeting where one or another key person was missing, so that a vote would not be called for. After a few months he decided to face the issue. In characteristic fashion he spent most of the afternoon on trivia but finally asked for a vote on my resignation. The swing vote was cast by Lyman, the professor of neuropsychiatry. We had had little contact and I was rather surprised.

During the period between my letter of resignation and my reinstatement, I continued my programs of teaching and research. The students, without any input on my part, petitioned Dave to keep me. The leader of this group, Suyd Osterhout, was a member of the Dean's family, a future chief resident in Medicine and an active member of the current Duke faculty. Fortunately for me, while the issue was in doubt I made no critical remarks about any member of my Department. I had come to Duke because of the strength and vigor of the clinical group. I had no deep philosophical issues to resolve.

In retrospect I can see a number of reasons why the medical faculty became so anxious. I had brought with me to Duke four young men, all destined for bright careers in academic medicine. I knew that they would all in due time leave Duke, and I wanted to give them as rich an experience as possible. I knew the senior clinicians at Duke performed well without me and that, because of their level of income, they would never go to another academic institution. I therefore, as a part of my educational program, assigned the new faculty members to run the Department and chair key committees when I was out of town. It never crossed my mind that this would create anxiety or resentment.

I had never taken myself very seriously and, in my first two years at Duke, I said whatever crossed my mind. I had grown up in medical schools where the clinical faculty were independent of the medical school. What the chairman said made little difference. They could always take their practice elsewhere. The situation at Duke was very different. All the established clinicians at Duke were totally dependent for their livelihood on Duke Hospital. What the chief of medicine said or did had a tremendous effect on their pocketbooks. They were attached to the University and medical school. They wanted acceptance as full-fledged faculty members. They did not want to be protected from teaching assignments or committee work because they were busy clinicians. They wanted the service arranged so that by working long hours they could give excellent service to patients and write scholarly papers based on their clinical experience. This deep attachment to Duke and the importance of the Department in the lives of its members was to be my greatest asset. I underestimated the intensity of the asset and in the beginning used it poorly.

The Executive Committee laid down one requirement: namely, that I put in writing an administrative plan which was acceptable to the Department of Medicine. This was worked out in a series of meetings between the staff and it has functioned successfully during the succeeding years.

The essence of the agreement was as follows:

1) The chairman of the Department would continue to request from the Dean $2,500 for each member of the Department.

2) All policies relating to teaching and patient care would be decided by majority vote of members of the Department with the rank of associate (not associate professor) or above.

3) The tax for research and teaching paid by the clinicians would be determined by a committee of four, elected by secret ballot. The chairman of the Department would chair this committee.

4) The chairman of the Department could use the private diagnostic clinic for partial support of any member of the Department. Whenever the income earned by the clinical activities of a member of the Department was projected to be above 50% of his total income, approval of a majority of the practicing staff was necessary.

5) Wayne Rundles would become a permanent member of the faculty.

The only issues that were different from my original projections were the retention of the small stipends from the portion of the money assigned to the Department by the Dean and the stabilization of Rundles' position in the Department. I had not made up my mind about him. His colleagues had accurately appraised his potential and he became one of my most valued colleagues.

I had undoubtedly created some anxiety in my colleagues by a series of actions:

1) I made aggressive moves to find space for departmental labora-

tories. I used the scientific knowledge of my research-minded clinicians to cover problems of clinical physiology and biochemistry. I brought in a clinician interested in infectious disease who established a laboratory not dependent on the Department of Bacteriology. These moves threatened the basic science areas. This seemed illogical to me because I was the clinical chairman most committed to their support. I was just learning that feeling states determine actions and that logic is usually irrelevant.

2) Ed Orgain was a superior teacher and clinician. His colleague was a liability. I obtained his resignation.

3) The neurologists required research and teaching funds created by the other clinicians for their basic support. They said that it was impossible for clinical neurologists to support themselves in a medical center. I never believed this and cut off their subsidy. The three neurologists left. Since that time clinical neurology has been a self-supporting division.

4) I eliminated the lecture series given by the clinical staff and opened up more time for teaching by the residents and fellows.

5) I put junior students in the clinic and senior students on the ward.

6) I promoted Walter Kempner to a full professorship. He was at that time not loved by all his colleagues.

It never occurred to me that the core of our excellent clinical staff would be concerned about my actions. They were the reason for my coming to Duke. Without them the place was insolvent and the future grim. With them, all of the things that I wanted to happen would happen.

David Smith and I had an interesting relationship. We started off on the wrong foot because he, the acting chairman of the Department, was away at the time of my appointment. This seemed like poor planning to me but I did not know until later that this had occurred.

I believed that Duke had become rather ingrown at the house staff level and I advised a number of our most able students to take their internship elsewhere. I broke up long-standing arrangements with the University of Rochester and the Hopkins, because I did not think they were sending us their best students. This approach did not endear me to Deryl Hart or David Smith.

From the beginning I had the good sense to appreciate that David Smith was one of the giants of the Duke medical school. I list him alongside Davison, Hart, Hanes and Beard. He had a foot in the basic science area as professor of bacteriology and a foot in the clinical service as associate professor of medicine and the man Dr. Hanes left in charge in his absence. He interpreted the clinician's problems to his basic science colleagues and the scientist's problems to the clinicians. He was interested in having a small, highly personalized department of bacteriology. This allowed him to obtain credibility as a person above the fray who was not contending for space or money. He brought wisdom to our deliberations. As the years went by, I discussed with him many problems and benefited by his wisdom. I'm proud to say that having started as a non-supporter of Stead he gradually became one of my strongest allies. [1977]

* * * *

By the time of my arrival at Duke in January 1947, it was obvious that Julian Ruffin was one of the iron men of the Duke medical school. He ran the medical outpatient clinic in an effortless way, operated an active program in the medical private diagnostic clinic and had plenty of time left over for thinking and clinical research. In those days, he always left Durham by driving to Virginia to catch the train. He recognized Duke University as a worthy competitor of "the University" (naturally, the University of Virginia), but he did not believe that trains had yet reached North Carolina!

Dr. Ruffin has always had many young men around him. His excellent clinical sense, his curiosity about the workings of the gastrointestinal tract, and his own willingness to pitch in and work have made his service both popular and productive. He has peopled the gastrointestinal world with his products. He is recognized now as a wise man who serves on a consultant basis to all groups seriously interested in gastroenterology. The National Institutes of Health and the Veterans Administration frequently call on him for advice and help. [1967]

* * * *

Traditionally, a department of medicine has the greatest impact on undergraduate teaching of any group in a medical school, and a review of the activities of our department makes the reasons for this clear. In gross anatomy, the incoming students meet Bill Knisely, who has a joint appointment in Anatomy and Medicine. Bill continues to see these students through the years as they feed back from the clinical years into his research program. In neuroanatomy in the first year, they are taught by Talmage Peele who also has a joint appointment in Anatomy and Medicine. On the wards in the third and fourth years, again they meet Talmage as he helps them take care of sick patients. He sees at first hand what part of his teaching is significant in the third and fourth years. As first-year students in biochemistry, they meet Bill Lynn in his work as a chemist concerned with the behavior of enzymes and steroids. In the third and fourth years, Bill sees patients with the students on the wards and in the diabetic clinic. In physiology, Frank Engel is responsible for the teaching of endocrinology.

He is also chairman of the committee which directs clinical endocrinology. The biological importance of recording cell potentials is covered by Harvey Estes who teaches cardiology in the clinical years. In the second year, David Smith, who holds the joint titles of professor of microbiology and associate professor of medicine, teaches bacteriology. For years he has worked with the third- and fourth-year students on clinical problems in the areas of fungus disease and tuberculosis. John Overman, with a primary appointment in bacteriology, covers the area of viruses and ricksettsia. He functions also as an assistant professor of medicine and handles clinical problems involving allergy and viruses. Suyd Osterhout, who is in charge of clinical bacteriology, teaches one quarter as a bacteriologist and three as an internist. In the second year, some 15 members of the department work with the students in introductory medicine covering history taking, physical diagnosis and clinical laboratory methods. In the third and fourth years, one-fourth of the student's time is spent in the Department of Medicine. In addition, many students work with us during their elective quarter and during summer vacations. [1959]

* * * *

I am 50 years old today and this has stimulated me to review the past and look into the future.

The past has been fun. I had the good fortune to be appointed professor of medicine at Emory University in 1942 at the age of 33. Many of my students have now reached full maturity and are leaders in the fields of teaching, clinical medicine and research. Our department has supplied academic leadership in many universities. Paul Beeson at Yale, Sam Martin at Gainesville, Jack Myers at Pittsburgh, John Hickam at Indiana, and Jim Warren at Galveston are chairmen of their respective departments of medicine and leaders in their medical schools. All have taken with them a contingent of Emory and Duke men, so that education in these five institutions has a real "Steadian" flavor.

Members of our department have gone on to leadership in other fields. Peritz Scheinberg is professor of neurology at Miami and Bernard Holland is professor of psychiatry at Emory University. Bill Knisely is going to the new school at Lexington, Kentucky as professor of anatomy.

Two weeks ago I met the dean of another medical school who is approaching Frank Engel for a department chairmanship, and next Saturday the associate dean of Stanford will be in Durham. He says he is looking for a Stead-trained professor of medicine. [1958]

•

Reversible "madness" is a syndrome which no doctor likes to miss. Many forms of reversible delirium are endocrine in origin. Dr. VanWyk's excellent article on hypothyroidism in this issue of *Medical Times* brings to mind my own interest in endocrine and other forms of reversible "madness".

Patients with delirium are seen on all services and their confusion may lead to weird tales. I remember well the lady from a North Carolina seashore town who became mad. She was urged by family and doctors to come to Duke Hospital but refused because she kept hearing strange noises. She finally consented to come if cotton were stuffed into her ear canals to keep out the sounds. The staff at Duke found her too deaf to examine properly and she was sent from the ward to the ear clinic. The ward had a new orderly and he took her, by error, to the eye clinic. The late Frank Engel, a very astute physician and endocrinologist, happened to take a short cut through the eye clinic, spotted the abnormal pigmentation and mental confusion and called the ward to find out how long their Addisonian patient had been delirious. The staff denied having a patient with adrenal insufficiency but, once alerted, quickly established the correctness of Dr. Engel's diagnosis and appropriate therapy cured the delirium.[3]

•

Frank [Engel] is one of the most brilliant people I have ever known. He has, in the last few years, become nationally recognized, and is now confronted with that familiar problem of how much to work at home and how much to speak abroad.

He is an excellent teacher and a fine doctor. Personally, I would hate for him to take a place which meant that he would see no more patients. My guess would be that a joint appointment, in physiology and medicine, would appeal to him more than one restricted entirely to physiology. [1951]

•

I am in the awkward situation of having to write as good a letter about Frank Engel as I did about John Hickam. It just so happens that this department does have a number of unusually able folk.

Frank is a person of wide interests and abilities. His research work has become internationally known and he is in great demand throughout the country on all types of metabolic and endocrinological projects. He is developing a fine resident and fellowship program in clinical endocrinology and metabolism. He is completely responsible for the administrative activities in his own unit and these responsibilities are handled effectively. [1956]

* * * *

Everyone who knew John Hickam comments on his incisive mind, the unusual breadth of his interests, the ability to explore new kinds of knowledge, the ability to see to the heart of a problem and bend other men's minds to his way of thinking. But John was more than a highly intelligent, well-organized performer. He had an unusual degree of humility, of whimsical humor, of tolerance and understanding which bound men to him and to his ventures. We do miss John Hickam. He always carried on when the going was tough. We will have to follow his example. [1970]

* * * *

Jack Myers has an extraordinary ability for the clear presentation of complicated data. He has developed an outstanding research program centered about the circulation and metabolism of the splanchnic regions. His studies have gone far to clarify this mysterious area. Even cursory reading of his publications demonstrates the depth of his thinking and his inherent ability for clear statement. His studies have required him to learn a large number of techniques and he is unusually competent with his hands.

Myers is a doctor's doctor. Students, residents and staff bring their personal problems and their family problems to him. [1951]

•

Jack Myers frequently said that much clinical learning could be summarized by the statement: any positive observation has greater weight than any negative observation. If a marble is found in a room, that is a positive observation and, in general, means that the room did contain a marble. If the doctor finds no marble on searching the room, it may mean that there is no marble there, but many times it will mean that the doctor is not good at finding marbles.

* * * *

Kempner's greatest triumphs came in the treatment of malignant hypertension. Here was a dramatic disease of short duration in which he could demonstrate reversibility. The outcome of the disease was well enough known so that the favorable effects could be reasonably attributed to diet. Patients who at that time would have died in all other hospitals had a reasonable chance for survival if they came under Kempner's care. The closing sentence of a talk which he gave 25 years ago to the 30th Annual Session of the American College of Physicians was as follows: "The important result is not that the change in the course of the disease has been achieved by the rice diet but that the course of the disease can be changed."

It is of interest to consider why Kempner has received in this country little recognition for his tremendous achievements. He did not appeal to the scientific community. It wanted him to set up various kinds of control studies. He contended that each patient was his own control and that there were already enough studies of patients treated by other forms of therapy. He was unwilling to deny any of his patients the full benefit of what he thought was best. Moreover, he pointed to his unequivocal results on rats with experimental hypertension, nephrosis and polyarteritis.

He has made many enemies because he has been honest and uncompromising and has never spent a single hour of his life, except for some scientific talks on rare occasions, in any society or even in a committee meeting. [1964]

•

The Kempner story is an interesting one. He was brought to Duke by Dr. Hanes to work on the metabolism of kidney cells. He believed that the clinicians could use some of the information that he had to help their patients with renal insufficiency. In essence he proposed a diet of rice and carbohydrates derived mostly from fruits. His clinical colleagues laughed at him. Dr. Hanes supported him and made available to him patients on the public ward. To everyone's surprise except Kempner, his patients did better than those of other members of the staff. No one referred any private patients to Kempner so Hanes opened up the private diagnostic clinic to him. He rapidly built a tremendous practice, caring for patients from all states in the union and from most foreign countries. Duke was a state and regional school until the advent of Kempner. He made Duke visible on the national and international scenes.

The senior clinicians at Duke did not admire Kempner and he was not always charitable in his comments about them. He was supported by David Smith who had refused to fire him during his term as acting chairman. I reviewed the charges against Kempner. They were primarily directed against his method of record keeping. His records consisted of a minimum of verbiage and a maximum of measurements to which a numerical value could be assigned. These records, though they seemed strange at the time, are very similar to those that we now find profitable to store in the hospital.

After a review of the situation, I decided that Kempner had the best records and the best followup of anyone in the institution. I checked the output of his laboratories and found the data of high quality. My recommendation was that Kempner be promoted to a full professorship.

Kempner and I enjoyed each other as persons and respected each other as persons and respected each other professionally. We did not always agree but we were wise enough to listen to each other. I knew that Kempner had a disciplined, well-trained and original mind. I negotiated with him more successfully than most because I never underestimated Kempner's intelligence. [1977]

•

Kempner has dedicated his life to the study of vascular disease and his strikes have all been made in areas where the experts said there was no gold. Who in his right mind would have ever thought that rice and fruit could modify vascular disease appreciably? Who would have fed a protein-deficient patient, losing large quantities of protein in his urine, a protein-poor diet? Who would have dared to give a more than 90% carbohydrate diet to a diabetic? Every expert knew that cholesterol levels were not influenced by diet. Nevertheless, all these leads have paid off richly. [1958]

* * * *

Deryl Hart was the toughest negotiator this school will ever have, and one can be certain that Surgery never came out with the short end of the stick. [1973]

* * * *

[To the Dean]: I would like for the new chairman of the department to have the same freedom to bring in new people and to make needed changes which I have had. For this reason, this projected change requires some careful financial planning. For the 10-year period from June 1968 to June 1978, the budget of the department will need to be increased by the amount of my salary. I am paid equally from University and departmental funds. By 1968, sufficient department funds will have accumulated during my tenure to cover my salary for a 10-year period. The University needs to make plans in advance for the portion of my salary carried by them.

The progress of the Medical Center can be greatly limited by intellectual failure of one of its major departmental heads. The best way for the University to insure itself against this potential hazard to its intellectual and financial security is to have the decisions in regard to long-range policy and in regard to new appointments to the staff in the hands of young men. If my health remains good, I will simply continue to work at whatever tasks I seem best suited for, and the University suffers no loss. If I become unable to function well and my colleagues wish to give me less work, the University does lose something. Its loss under this arrangement is small compared to the loss if I should remain as chairman under these conditions.

I therefore present this program to the University as a form of insurance which will assure the continued excellence of that area in the medical school which has been entrusted to my care. [1960]

•

[To Harvard Dean]: I have made the decision to accept the Commonwealth's offer to use their facilities as my base of operations for 1968. I lived in Boston in the days of my youth. I'd better leave my memories untainted by reality and the cold light of more advanced years. I am both pleased and honored that you would have been willing to arrange a year at Harvard. [1967]

•

Your editor [EAS] has many enthusiasms. He is moved by the excitement of the times. By nature he spends most of his time working for the things that move him; by nature too, he is more apt to express himself as *for* than *against*. He is *for* the new Duke medical school curriculum which allows the medical student to become a clinical clerk in June after he enters medical school in September. He is *not against* other curricula. He is *for* the development of assistants recruited and trained by the doctor and capable of extending the doctor's arms, hands and brain. He is *not against* the recruiting and training of other personnel by non-physicians. He is *for* the intelligent structuring of groups for effective practice and continuing education. He is *not against* solo practice. He is *for* making more available complex laboratory tests and reducing their unit cost by greater use. He is *not against* the best use of the history and physical examination.[7]

* * * *

[*New Rules*]: Beginning with the 1972 meeting, a registration fee will be charged all who attend meetings of the American Federation for Clinical Research, American Society for Clinical Investigation and Association of American Physicians. The registration fee will be $15 for all members and non-members, except that students, house officers and fellows will be charged only $10, for which they will receive the abstracts without payment of the regular $6 cost. The registration fee will be the same for attendance of one or all three of the sequential meetings.

The members of the Council of the Association of American Physicians regret the passing of the old days and wish that these steps did not have to be taken. Realistically, we believe they do. [*Written in 1971 as president of Association of American Physicians*]

•

I envisage that within my lifetime (I appear rather healthy), the first quarter of medical school, or the bridge periods between the college and medical school, will be devoted to learning how to handle the problems of information and to prepare each student to have a stake in clinical epidemiology.

Just one more personal note. I am still an active teacher of clinical students and house staff. I edit *Circulation* and I take care of 325 aging folk. I am chairman of the committee which integrates the medical information systems that we are developing in the Medical Center and has the responsibility for interrelating these systems used by the doctors with the IBM systems now becoming operational at Duke Medical Center. Life remains both pleasant and active. [1977]

* * * *

[*To Medcom Editor*]: I appreciate the time and thought you spent in editing my manuscript. This is a rather personal venture, and I have a style of speaking and writing which is well known to a number of generations of students at many levels. I would prefer to keep my somewhat idiomatic approach rather than use your changes which, in terms of projecting anyone but myself, are obvious improvements.

* * * *

One matter of history. I never took the Boards of internal medicine for two reasons: a) I was too poor, and b) I did not like the emphasis on formal training. All of the leaders in any new field came into leadership with a minimum of formal training. Then they set up a very formal program. For the majority of persons these programs are simpler and easier than the "do it yourself" approach. In any individual instance, the informal approach may be excellent.

* * * *

Bess Cebe and I have worked together since October 1951. When she is at work I seem to the outside world to be well organized, competent and efficient. When she is away on vacation or when she had her one prolonged illness, I appeared disorganized, forgetful, distracted, and inefficient.

Bess organizes my day, decides how long I spend at each task, makes all appointments, and softens my somewhat crusty appearance. She is the friend and confidante of generations of students, house staff, young faculty, secretaries and technicians.

Bess has a quick retentive mind and a liking for figures. She handled all of the grants during my tenure as chairman and had a hand in drafting of most research proposals. Because of her wide experience she has become a medical school resource. An amazingly large number of persons call on her for all types of information.

Bess has one very unusual quality which has made her nearly unique. She can be repetitively interrupted and not lose her train of thought or her train of figures. She tells me that she is not quite as unmoved by interruptions as she used to be. I cannot, however, detect any falling off in this unusual gift.

Bess did by herself an amount of work that normally is done by several people. She accomplished this by her quick mind, her well-organized schedule, and an ability to administer and to type accurately and rapidly. She started when the department was still small and therefore had the advantage of knowing the origin and purpose of all the divisions and the details of their budget. The new chairman had to quadruple his staff when Bess moved out of the chairman's office to take care of me and of the Myocardial Infarction Research Unit.

Bess had the ability to accept the virtues and liabilities of a young and aggressive staff. She liked us even though she recognized our weaknesses. She skillfully accentuated our strengths and minimized our liabilities. She did all this without hostility or anger.

Bess was widowed during World War II. I enjoyed watching her raise her one child, Pete. She loved him, cared for him, disciplined him and, when he was full grown, turned him over to a wife without resentment. She has a collection of Pete's paintings which we call "early Cebes". They are the envy of all of us with less gifted children.

Bess likes men and they like her, I have watched a series of men who hoped that she would marry them and be cared for by her. She has enjoyed her own life too much to give it up for a mere male. She continues to enjoy both men and her freedom.

I have been fortunate in being surrounded by competent people all of my life. I have always had the "troops" to support any venture that I wished to undertake. This office can produce a complex application in an unbelievably short time. Bess must, of course, do the final work while at the end I only have to sign my name. In the final hours of a rushed up job, I am her assistant: carrying messages, running the copying machine, pushing the office of research grants to sign off in their area, and getting the right number of stamps for the mailing. We are indeed an effective team! [1977]

* * * *

This is the first generation in which the majority of persons between 40 and 60 years of age are financially responsible for three generations. Each family with children has at least four grandparents and, in this day and age, at least one of the grandparents will survive and become partially or completely senile. This last week I have been shopping for a very sweet but beginning-to-be confused grandmother. She is used to doing for herself and she does not adapt easily to having other people do for her. She tells her house-helper not to do most things. She intends to do them herself. But alas, she forgets and they are never done. She likes the visiting nurse who helps her with personal cleanliness and gives her advice about cooking,

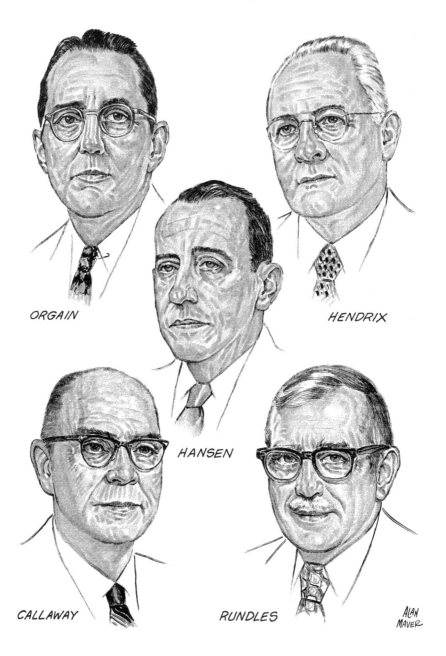

Senior Staff, Duke Department of Medicine, 1947

eating and shopping but, again, she cannot believe that she can't go it on her own.

As I shopped in the community where she has spent her life, I found good will on all sides. The saleswoman in the department store, the assistant manager of the bank, the salesmen responsible for mattresses, pillows and linens were interested in my problem: how to keep my lady functioning and living in her community. Each of them has faced similar problems. They look on the nursing home as inevitable but each, on the basis of his own experience, hopes that that time can be postponed. They have no good answers to old age, nor do I.

What shall we do if Grandmother slips and breaks her hip? What shall we do if she develops pneumonia? Must medical science intervene and keep her breathing but not living?

Our family must face the problem and advise Grandmother's doctor of our feelings. We as parents must remember that the patterns we devise for our parents are likely to be followed by our children when they must make similar decisions.

Many years ago, I wrote my own personal physician a letter to guide his hand if I became ill and my mind was not functioning normally. I quote from that letter:

"If I become ill and unable to manage my own affairs, I want you to be responsible for my care. To make matters as simple as possible, I will leave certain specific instructions with you.

"In event of unconsciousness from an automobile accident, I do not wish to remain in a hospital for longer than two weeks without full recovery of my mental faculties. While I realize that recovery might still be possible, the risk of living without recovery is still greater. At home, I want only one practical nurse. I do not wish to be tube-fed or given intravenous fluids at home.

"In the event of a cerebral accident, other than a subarachnoid hemorrhage, I want no treatment of any kind until it is clear that I will be able to think effectively. This means no stomach tube and no intravenous fluids.

"In the event of a subarachnoid hemorrhage, use your own judgment in the acute stage. If there is considerable brain damage, send me home with one practical nurse.

"If, in spite of the above care, I become mentally incapacitated and have remained in good physical condition, I do not want money spent on private care. I prefer to be institutionalized, preferably in a state hospital.

"If any other things happen, this will serve as a guide to my own thinking.

"Go ahead with an autopsy with as little worry to my wife as possible."

Now the time has come to write a letter to Grandmother's doctor. He is a wise man and will appreciate the support a family can give in a problem for which there is no wholly satisfactory answer.[8]

REFERENCES

1. Stead EA. J. Clin. Invest. **32**: 548, 1953.
2. Stead EA. Medical Times **94**: 1250, 1966.
3. Stead EA. Medical Times **94**: 1404, 1966.
4. Stead EA, Interview. Modern Medicine, August 1958, p. 175.
5. Stead EA. Arch. Int. Med. **133**: 756, 1974.
6. Stead EA. Am. J. Diseases Child. **124**: 343, 1972.
7. Stead EA. Medical Times **94**: 370, 1966.
8. Stead EA. Medical Times **98**: 191, 1970.

PART III
Recollections

11

Eugene Anson Stead, Jr.: An Appreciation*

JOHN B. HICKAM, M.D.

The Grady Hospital of 25 years ago was not a likely place to start raising a family of medical scholars, and the fact that it was done there shows the extraordinary talent of the man who did the job.

How did Eugene Stead go about doing this job and others like it in later years? In the first place, this teacher had, even in the early years, reasonably good material to work with, and this was no accident. He drew good people to him. Later on, good people were attracted in part by seeing that things went well for those who had worked with Stead, but in the beginning they had to be attracted largely by their own estimate of the man. What are some of the qualities that proved so attractive to critical, ambitious young people even in the days when the professor himself was very young? Of course he was, and is, himself critical, ambitious and competitive, although now more urbane in the display of these characteristics than he was 25 years ago. He was even then an outstandingly competent clinician, and this always commands the respect of pupils young and old. He was a skilled clinical investigator who was doing exciting and imaginative work in the field of cardiovascular disease, but such an attribute mainly draws people who know already that they want to do the same kind of work, and most of us had no such definite ideas in mind when we first joined Stead.

He was hard-working and demanded that others work hard too, but this trait by itself has only a limited power to attract pupils. He demanded excellence in all professional activities. He believed in himself, had faith in his own judgment, and enjoyed watching his own head work on a problem. These are attractive and interesting traits if the judgment and the head are good enough, which they were.

While all these comments are true, they do not begin to explain the

*Ann. Int. Med. 69: 993, 1968

peculiarly compelling effect that Stead exerted on the young men around him. They wanted very much to deserve his good opinion and not to merit his disapproval. When he first moved to Duke there was a sinister charac- ter in the comic strips called "Influence" who bent people to his will by a hypnotic stare from his prominent green eyes. We who remained at Emory were soon charmed with the news that medical students—and others—at Duke had begun to call Dr. Stead "Influence". How could he have such an effect on tough-minded, independent young people? We too were critical, ambitious, competitive and, in our own private judgments, fine clinicians, skilled investigators either actually or potentially, and hard-working men dedicated to excellence. How did he get to us?

This is one of the crucial questions in trying to understand a great teacher. What does he show that alerts people to his special presence? This probably has different answers for different pupils. For many of us, the most attractive and compelling intellectual feature of Dr. Stead has always been his tremendous ability to analyze a complicated problem, reduce it to essentials, and express it with clarity. When one puts this ability together with a strong and determined character, a gift for colorful statement, and the other traits I have already mentioned, then a picture does begin to emerge of a teacher, a service chief, a senior research partner, and an administrator who commanded deep respect and whose good opinion was earnestly desired.

The skill and the response have depended in large part on the consistent, devoted use of his talents to enhance the understanding and development of pupils.

Stead students know the phrase, "Life is hard". It became famous from situations in which a complex medical problem of the night before would be described, with a detailed account of herculean diagnostic and therapeutic efforts. After Dr. Stead had heard about the problem for a while, he would ask for additional data as, for instance, "What did the spinal fluid show?" The unfortunate house officer, who now perceived that it would indeed have been useful to know about the spinal fluid but did not have the information, would still be anxious to defend his position. "Dr. Stead", he would say, "we were up until four o'clock with this patient, and it was a very confusing picture at the time, and we did all these other tests, and so on". This was the point at which the axe would fall: "What you're telling me is that life is hard. I already know that. What I want to know is, what did the spinal fluid show?"

Bedside medicine provided rich opportunities to show the value of clearly identifying and examining the basic findings and assumptions that were being used to understand and manage a puzzling illness. Many a pupil's embarrassment began with the words, "I think this patient is trying to tell us something"; or the harsher criticism that came when the professor was convinced that nobody was getting an effective message from the sick man: "What this patient needs is a doctor!"

Stead's remarkable ability to think clearly and freshly has helped pupils to deal successfully with many different kinds of problems. Years ago one of his young professors who was a new department chairman elsewhere complained of his frustration and unhappiness because the administration of his school seemed indecisive, aimless, and slow to move. Gene could have said simply, "Life is hard". What he did say was, "A strong, decisive administration is helpful to you only if their ideas happen to coincide with yours. Otherwise, it's much better to have an administration that will leave you alone, and then you can work things out for yourself".

He paid close attention to his pupils and so came to understand them individually very well. He was determined to make them grow. To this end he often gave jobs to people who needed to grow when others could have done the work better. He removed his name from many scientific papers written by pupils who were working out his ideas. For those who did not respond to his efforts, he had little time because there were many pupils. In those who did respond, he built confidence, self-respect, a conviction of being on the first team, and a need to live up to that position that carried them where they otherwise would not have gone.

He has helped us to understand, to grow up, and to do what we can do. We bear some scars, but we are very grateful.

12

Eugene A. Stead, Jr.: A Biographical Note*

PAUL B. BEESON, M.D.

I first became acquainted with Gene Stead in 1939 at the Peter Bent Brigham Hospital where he was a research fellow in medicine. Before that, he had spent his boyhood in Atlanta and had studied medicine at Emory. After internships in both medicine and surgery at the Brigham he had gone to the Thorndike Laboratories as research fellow, then to the Cincinnati General Hospital where he was chief resident in Medicine. He had returned to the Thorndike for a year; then moved to the Brigham when his chief, Soma Weiss, at age 39, became Hersey Professor of the Theory and Practice of Medicine at Harvard and Physician-in-Chief to the Brigham Hospital. Weiss liked young people and gave them scope. One of my first impressions on taking up my residency there was to note with some surprise that comparatively young doctors were pushed to the fore and that they could be stimulating and exciting teachers. Weiss gave such men as Stead and Charles Janeway, both research fellows, regular turns as attending physicians on the medical wards. The word soon got around among students and house officers that their rounds were among the best.

I visited the ward where Stead was attending one day and can recall the scene with great clarity. He had been shown a man just admitted with hemiplegia after a cerebrovascular accident. In examining the patient Stead noted that he had edema that was unilateral in distribution. He turned to the group accompanying him and for about half an hour led a discussion of the probable mechanism of this phenomenon. Subsequently, I saw him do that sort of thing many times. He was truly fascinated by the mechanism of pathologic events. In addition, he enjoyed the challenge of having to find some noteworthy aspect of a case that others might have passed off as a common and rather uninteresting clinical problem.

*Ann. Int. Med. 69: 968, 1968

In 1942, at the age of 33, Stead was invited to return to Emory as its first fulltime Professor of Medicine. It was my good fortune to be invited to go along in the only other fulltime post in the department. He also took with him from Harvard James Warren as research fellow and John Hickam as resident in Medicine. In Atlanta we shared the teaching and patient care with a group of able physicians in practice there, and for the next four years at Grady Hospital, all of us experienced a truly exciting adventure in medicine. Those years saw the first clinical trials of penicillin; in research, there was the introduction of the flame photometer and the cardiac catheter. Our grand rounds on Sunday mornings drew packed audiences: students, house officers, local physicians and medical officers from nearby military hospitals.

In research Stead forged a remarkably effective partnership with Warren. They were invited by the Office of Scientific Research and Development to undertake a study of shock, using the "new" technique of cardiac catheterization. Warren spent some time at Bellevue Hospital learning the methods from Drs. Cournand and Richards, then he and Stead set up their own laboratory adjacent to the emergency department at Grady. They used this special laboratory to the full, not only in the study of shock but to obtain information about many other cardiovascular matters. Their laboratory, together with that of McMichael in London, did much to define normal values and to measure the effects of anxiety and postural changes. Their work on the influence of anemia on circulatory dynamics is still referred to. They explored the use of the catheter in other parts of the circulatory system, finding that they could obtain samples from the pulmonary arteries as well as the hepatic and renal veins. Their brief notes announcing these were the first in the field. This team was also the first to make use of the technique of cardiac catheterization as an aid to diagnosis of congenital heart disease.

While waiting in the emergency department of the hospital for shock patients to come in at night, Stead, Warren and their colleagues, Arthur Merrill and Emmett Brannon, held long discussions of the physiology of the cardiovascular system and of the sequence of pathologic events in circulatory disorders. Stead and Warren tested some of this thinking with careful observations of patients in heart failure and eventually formulated a "forward failure" hypothesis. The hypothesis, supported by comparatively little in the way of tabular information, was published in their celebrated "fluid dynamics" paper. This aroused great interest and no little controversy, centering on the stark opening sentence in the conclusions: "Edema develops in chronic congestive failure because the kidneys do not excrete salt and water in a normal manner".

In 1946 Stead was invited to take the chairmanship of the Department of Medicine at Duke. To those of us associated with him at Emory, things were going so well that the thought of his leaving was almost inconceivable; nevertheless, he did decide to move. Undoubtedly a factor was that he had found the additional administrative burden irksome. Another was that he saw the immense advantages in the situation at Duke, where the hospital was under university control and where there was a completely flexible system of faculty appointments, ranging from fulltime private practice to fulltime academic work. As I have struggled with such matters subsequently in other places, I have often recalled how quickly he appreciated, and later made good use of, the possibilities presented at Duke. So off he went.

In the next 20 years at Duke, Stead built up a large and outstanding Department of Medicine, making the fullest use of the flow of public and private benefactions into medical research and teaching. A Veterans Hospital was constructed on the campus, and he smoothly moved people back and forth between that and the University hospital. Always he tended to put young people into positions of responsibility and somehow managed to help them bear responsibility ably. With all the growth, the recruitment and the necessary traveling, he gradually found it necessary to give up personal participation in research but continued to be in close touch with what the other members of his department were doing, frequently displaying that characteristic knack of recognizing something of interest in the findings that others had overlooked. One portion of a professor's work that he never allowed to shrink was active participation in teaching and patient care. Never was there a doubt that the man at the top was a good doctor or that he placed a high value on clinical performance.

Stead is relinquishing the chairmanship of his department several years before the statutory retirement age. He will continue to work there and will of course go on with the teaching of clinical medicine, not only at home but in many other schools, because he is justly recognized as the unmatchable visiting professor. I predict that he will develop a new career activity, plunging into that as if a second stage rocket had ignited, putting him in a different orbit. Of late he has become increasingly concerned about problems of delivering good medical services to all the people, and this may be the area to which he will give his major attention. That would be everyone's good fortune, because he is a wise man.

13

The Original Department of Medicine at Duke and The Arrival of Dr. Stead As Chairman

DRS. J.L. CALLAWAY, E.S. ORGAIN, J.M. RUFFIN AND D.T. SMITH

In February 1977, GSW arranged for meetings of Drs. Callaway, Orgain, Ruffin and D.T. Smith to record their memories of this subject. The following is a transcription of those meetings.

David T. Smith, Professor Emeritus of Medicine and Microbiology: President Few had contacted Dr. Welch, who was the original dean at the Johns Hopkins Medical School, and asked for his help in finding a dean to organize the Duke medical school. Dr. Welch recommended Dr. Wilburt Davison who was at that time assistant dean of the medical school at Hopkins. Dr. Davison's selections for the faculty of the Duke medical school were made primarily from men already known and active at Hopkins. Dr. Davison selected Dr. Amoss as the professor of medicine, Dr. Hart as professor of surgery, and those two selected Dr. Carter as Ob-Gyn professor, Dr. Forbus for pathology, Dr. Swett for anatomy, and Dr. Eadie for physiology. I was invited down by Dr. Davison who said they had two jobs at the new medical school they thought I might fill. One was associate professor of medicine in charge of infectious diseases under Dr. Amoss and the other was an independent job as professor of bacteriology. After thinking for a few minutes, I said, 'Well, how about me taking both jobs?' Dr. Davison said, 'Oh, well now, there won't be but one pay', and so my next question was, 'Well, which pay is the best?' He said, 'Well, professor of bacteriology, of course, and you won't get any pay for being an associate professor of medicine.' I said, 'OK, that suits me fine.' And so under those conditions I filled these positions as primarily a bacteriologist but as the second man in the Department of Medicine.

When the medical school first opened, there was one ward for private medical patients and one for private surgical patients, the other wards all being public patients. But as the depression grew worse, there were fewer and fewer private patients, so that by 1930 there were not quite enough patients, really, to fill one ward. At this time, Dr. Hart began to try to devise some better financial method of attracting patients to the hospital. It happened that Dr. Amoss had gone to China for six months to the Peking medical school, and I was acting chairman of the Department of Medicine. So I was consulted on this plan. Dr. Hart felt that we ought to establish a private diagnostic clinic where patients could come in and have their diagnostic work for whatever they could afford to pay. This was a revolutionary idea and he sold it to Davison and to me. Then we called in all the staff that would be involved. Somewhat to our surprise, their vote was 50 for and 50 against. The meeting was postponed for 24 hours. The next day it was almost unanimous; but there is a fair possibility that, if Amoss had been here—since he never agreed with Hart or Davison on anything else—he would have opposed it and the diagnostic clinic would have never been established. But that is pure speculation.

Shortly after Amoss came back, his relationships with Davison became practically impossible. So Davison felt that Amoss would have to leave. I sat in on the meeting where the chiefs of all the departments were involved and defended Amoss to the best of my ability. His scientific background was excellent and he was a good teacher, but I could not break down the obvious evidence from all the departments that he was not a good co-operater. I did not vote against Dr. Amoss, since I was associate professor of medicine, but the others all voted against him. I took the occasion of this meeting, however, to say that since Davison had chosen to consult the department heads about dismissing Amoss instead of doing it on his own as dean, he had set a precedent for having all important decisions made by the department heads.

Dr. Frederic Hanes succeeded Amoss as professor of medicine. Hanes had been very well trained and had spent some of his time under Dr. Osler. He had had additional time in pathology and in neurology. After his training, he had returned to practice in Winston-Salem because of some family connections there. Hanes had not had any significant teaching experience but had a very good head for business. He organized the financial aspects of the department. First he started the Anna H. Hanes Fund which was a grant from his mother. This was supplemented by a taxation plan by which the medical staff with PDC incomes were reviewed each year by Hanes and me regarding their research activities and their teaching load. Decisions were relatively arbitrary and percent of taxation ranged from 5% to 20%. Hanes realized that the Department of Medicine was not doing well financially under the single PDC setup. Even though the fees for consultations were low throughout the medical center, the surgeons got additional money from their surgical procedures. This led to the separation of the medical and surgical PDC, with each having its own business manager and a different approach to the distribution of its financial income. Clarence Cobb became the first business manager of the medical private diagnostic clinic. This separation was accomplished by Hanes and Hart without the patients being aware of any change.

Edward S. Orgain, Professor Emeritus of Medicine: From the time of his appointment as professor and chairman of the Department of Medicine, Dr. Hanes gradually built up the staff of the department in an autocratic but benign way, and the department was run as a benign dictatorship, with Hanes as the central figure. He had easy access to Davison and to various succeeding presidents of the University who respected his thoughts and judgments and who gave him full backing.

Having suffered with hypertension during his later years when present-day drug therapy was not available, he developed a dissecting aneurysm of the thoracic aorta which ruptured three months after its inception and terminated in his death at the age of 63.

Following this, a search committee was appointed by Dr. Davison, with William M. Nicholson as chairman, to find a new chairman for the Department. Meanwhile, the Department was more or less directed by a committee of three: Drs. Smith, Ruffin and Callaway. They made the general decisions about the department, its appointments, its finances, and the running of the medical private diagnostic clinic, until the advent of Dr. Stead.

About 1947 the Dean, at the suggestion of the search committee, offered the chairmanship to Dr. Stead who was at that time professor of medicine and dean of the School of Medicine at Emory. Upon Stead's arrival, he interviewed the various members of the department and the resignation of only one member was requested. Blanket resignations were neither requested nor offered.

One of his first problems, which he laughingly admitted later, was the fact that he had never requested to see where the interns were quartered. Actually, their previous quarters on the third floor had been turned over to Psychiatry and the interns had rooms on the campus, but there were no on-call rooms close to the wards. For Dr. Stead's inspection, several on-call rooms were hastily remodeled for this purpose.

He then turned his attention toward the reorganization of teaching within the department, so that for the first time all private patients were assigned to students as well as to house officers. Regular rounding and teaching schedules were then maintained on a daily basis as they had been on the medical public wards for years. Patient acceptance of medical student workups and professional attention was indeed excellent, but the assistant resident on the private service often considered himself as a fifth-wheel man who did a great deal or little, depending on his attitude and his energies. Dr. Stead confessed to me privately that he knew how to run a ward service but he did not know how to run a private service and welcomed all suggestions. The use of the private services offered a tremendous amount of teaching material for students, interns, residents and particularly for fellows who were undergoing specialty training in various areas, notably cardiology.

Dr. Smith: The other important item in the development of the medical school was the introduction of Dr. Kempner who initiated his rice diet of low sodium and low cholesterol. They really were ward patients and they did very well while they were in the hospital under this restricted diet, but immediately relapsed when they went home. Hanes recognized that the medical patients would have to be a little more cooperative, and he asked the staff to refer some of their private patients to Kempner. They cooperated by referring hospital employees and members of the ministry and their families, who they would not have charged anyway. These patients did very well. But after Hanes discovered they were not going to voluntarily transfer paying patients to Kempner, he gave Kempner privilege of having his own patients. After Kempner's first paper was published, patients began to come from the whole United States and Kempner's income became the largest of the medical staff. At this point, Hanes started a heavy tax on Kempner for the benefit of the Anna H. Hanes Fund. After Stead was selected as Hanes' successor, Davison sent Dr. Ruffin out to my house with the message that I was to fire Kempner before Stead came to Duke. I sent back the message to Davison that I would not because it would not be fair to Kempner or to Stead, who was a heart specialist himself. He could determine whether he wanted to keep Kempner or not. Stead spent days reviewing x-rays and histories of Kempner's patients and decided to keep him.

With the diagnostic clinic operation at full speed and the Anna H. Hanes Fund, Stead had the most desirable chair of medicine in the United States and probably the whole world. He offered me a continuation of my appointment as associate professor of medicine without salary but with PDC privileges. Having served as an associate professor of medicine under Amoss and Hanes, I offered my advice when requested provided that he took it with his own risk that I was wrong.

Julian M. Ruffin, Professor Emeritus of Medicine: Dr. Stead, unlike Dr. Hanes, had a very strong background in teaching. Therefore, he spent a great deal of his time teaching the house staff and medical students.

J. Lamar Callaway, James B. Duke Professor of Dermatology: He immediately took over the job as professor and chairman of the department, and unobtrusively but enthusiastically let it be known that this was one of the two major services in this hospital and it was not going to be pushed around for space, for funds, or for recognition and, from the outset, he stood up to Hart, Davison and the other people, representing the Department of Medicine at the highest level of efficiency.

He might appear on the wards at any hour of day or night. He seemed to never show any evidence of fatigue and for the first few years he had a tendency to drive his staff and house staff in much the same fashion, believing unquestionably that no one had to die.

As the years passed, he mellowed considerably, realizing that there were some people who, in spite of 24-hour a day medical care under the best circumstances, could not survive; but in his early years, I don't believe he would accept this.

Dr. Ruffin: During Stead's first year as chairman, he did relatively little to change the department. He depended almost solely on his "brain trust" for consultation: Drs. Myers, Hickam and Engel.

Dr. Smith: I do recall on one occasion when he consulted me about capturing the basic $2,500 from the salary of his teaching staff and hiring another fulltime instructor. I objected to this on the grounds that the $2,500 was in recognition of their acceptance as a part of the University. I suggested that he could easily take an average of $5,000 from practicing staff PDC income if more funds were needed. He chose to continue to pursue the $2,500 salary. It became obvious to the whole school that the medical department was in trouble. Dr. Davison looked into the matter and called a special meeting of the Executive Committee. Stead refused to be ordered by the Committee as to how he ran his department. Finally he said, 'I will not be ordered but, if the matter is dropped, I will run the department in a manner that you will approve.' I said we had better accept this because he had given us a blank check for his dismissal if we don't approve. The changes made in the department were very remarkable, and the department ran smoothly from that time on.

Dr. Orgain: Following this, the Department at its regular monthly meetings made policy and other decisions by essentially majority vote of the members of the Department rather than by unilateral decision of the chairman. This arrangement worked out greatly to the advantage of the chairman, since any policy decision affecting the medical center and given to the Dean or the Executive Committee was always the voice of the Department of Medicine, not that of a single man.

Dr. Ruffin: It was only after the resolution of the problem concerning the University funds that those who had been in the department prior to

Stead's arrival began to feel they were part of the decision-making process. I feel that the money which the University had supplied to each of the departmental members was very important in the final establishment of TIAA-CREF. Under Hanes, there had been no full professors except the chairman. Soon after the resolution of the problem regarding the University funds, Stead promoted many of the more established men to full professor status. They had relatively little contact with Stead. He allowed them free rein in their areas but required that they generate the funds for supporting their areas. Thus each service was able to develop independently under Dr. Stead.

Dr. Callaway: Although primarily a cardiologist, he recognized and defended other subspecialties and never once in the 20 years I knew him as chairman did he fail to support the area of dermatology to the fullest extent that it deserved.

He was never too busy to give me an audience when I needed it and, when I asked for suggestions or advice, he gave me what I soon learned was always good sound, sage advice.

Although he was never the country club type, in my home he was a delightful guest and in his home he was a gracious host. I served with him on promotion committees, finance committees and other policy areas and, to my knowlege, he has never attempted to persuade me against my better judgment and at the same time he fought tooth and nail for all of medicine and its subspecialties in any area that he could.

When he came to Duke he told me he was going to retire after 20 years and he did.

Years Of Growth

Robert E. Whalen, m.d.*

A careful and balanced documentation of the achievements, failure, triumphs and tragedies encompassed in the years between Dr. Stead's arrival at Duke and his retirement as chairman of the Department of Medicine must await a careful and dispassionate analysis by a medical historian. It is not my intent to attempt such a project, both because of personal biases and because sufficient time has not elapsed to provide a truly objective evaluation of his era. Rather, I will attempt to provide an overview of Dr. Stead's philosophy, operating style, and impact on his department and the people he trained at Duke. My observations and conclusions stem from a multitude of experiences during my years as a house officer and a young faculty member. They represent a personal but hopefully not an individual interpretation of an era. I have labored to make them fair. They are less likely to be totally objective.

While those in the medical world who do not know him well address him as Dr. Stead and his peers address him as Gene, his young men called him Stead, when not within earshot. Although in later years he was Gene to me and to many of his house officers, he still is referred to as Stead in the many stories about him which inevitably flow when Stead-trained physicians gather. Thus, in this essay I will refer to him as Stead which to countless house officers and students conjures up memories of a man of wisdom, kindness, power, uncompromising honesty, and occasionally chilling ire.

Duke At The Beginning of the Stead Era

In order to understand the activity and the eventual effects of Stead's work in the Department of Medicine it is necessary to describe the forces

*Professor of Medicine and Chief, Cardiovascular Service, Duke; former house officer and chief resident, Duke Hospital.

operating in American medicine and in the Department of Medicine at Duke when he arrived in 1947. The country was emerging from a war which had mobilized all of its resources to provide the people and the materiel to win the war. In many ways academic medicine was emerging from a period of dormancy. Most medical centers had operated through the war years with a skeleton faculty which had worked itself to the bone training medical students 12 months a year. This mission often left the faculties so physically and intellectually exhausted that many of a medical center's traditional academic activities, such as vigorous research programs as well as more leisurely scholarly pursuits, had to be laid aside. The large scale research efforts that had been launched in the medical schools were primarily directed toward meeting the needs of a nation geared for war. Duke had participated in the traditional fashion in meeting the country's war needs. It had sent a hospital unit to Europe which depleted its faculty. Left behind was a cadre of extremely dedicated men who had not only taken on almost superhuman educational responsibilities but who also had maintained a large service responsibility to the region. Duke had handled its teaching responsibilities by relying heavily on the didactic approach, only because it provided the most efficient method of delivering information to students in an accelerated teaching schedule. All this was to change when Stead came.

When Stead arrived at Duke there were forces abroad in medicine and government which significantly changed medical education and practice. A veritable storehouse of new techniques and concepts had been generated by the demands of the national war effort. Physicians returned from military service with a thirst for more specialized knowledge of enlarging specialties in medicine. Furthermore, advanced training in medicine which had been relatively uncommon for a majority of physicians in the country became financially feasible because of personal savings generated during military service and government educational programs such as the GI Bill. Finally, the government rapidly assumed a majority role in financing postgraduate and research programs.

These were the vital ingredients present at the time of Stead's arrival at Duke. They were not clearly perceived by many when he came and much of his later success as an educator and a trainer of research workers stemmed from the fact that he did clearly understand the impact that these nascent forces would eventually have.

In a perhaps too simplistic way Stead's tenure as chairman of the Department of Medicine may be broken down into two eras. The first era, dating from 1947 when he arrived, lasted for approximately 12 years. Stead eventually brought with him from Emory four men who were to become giants in their own right in post-World War II American medicine. These lieutenants were John Hickam, who was later to become chairman of the Department of Medicine at Indiana, Jim Warren, who was later to become chairman of the Department of Medicine at the University of Texas in Galveston and then at Ohio State, Jack Myers who was later to become chairman of the Department of Medicine at the University of Pittsburgh, and Frank Engel, who died prematurely in 1963 while still at Duke. Although each was vastly different in personality, they all brought with them a thriving interest in clinical research and a total commitment to the vigorous teaching concepts of Stead. They complemented in a unique way the already strong clinical faculty that had emerged at Duke after the second world war. They were the cornerstones on which laboratory ventures were launched and they were the inspirational leaders in the recruitment of young people to research areas. Long before they left Duke, between 1954 and 1958, they had established themselves as leaders in American medicine. During the 10 to 12 years that they were at Duke they provided the leadership and the drawing power for a whole new crop of young people who were more laboratory oriented and who would eventually take their places as clinical investigators at Duke and other institutions.

The second era followed the departure of these strong men. By this time Stead had stocked his department well with young and ambitious people and, although most major departments of medicine could not stand to lose four outstanding men such as these in a very short period of time, Stead's department barely lost a stride. The young men left behind had been well prepared to take on responsibilities, both in the teaching and research area. Fortunately by this time public funding had become so abundant that it was relatively easy to find support for young people who had not yet made their name in the research area. Now this generation of young men has graduated to the gray-haired stage and many have been recruited away to other institutions but the principle of training a large stock of capable people who are always ready to step into a vacant position had been firmly established and funded so that the department has been left in as strong a position as it ever was.

Stead And The Private Diagnostic Clinic (PDC)

When Stead arrived from Atlanta the department already had a small cadre of extremely capable clinicians who had managed to maintain a large practice through the war years. Members of the private diagnostic clinic derived almost all their income from their own professional efforts. They received small salaries from the University primarily as a token of recognition that they were University faculty members. A portion of the income from this practice had traditionally been allocated to the chairman for his use in developing a research program. Although Stead wished to make changes within this PDC group he readily recognized that this source of income would be his venture capital for the future. He knew that the ability to generate private dollars was an invaluable asset. When he wanted to start a pilot project or finance a young man in a new venture he had the potential wherewithal to do this through the funds which were allocated to the chairman from the professional fees generated in the private diagnostic clinic.

Stead further recognized that you cannot have this type of system without motivation, and while he taxed the professional income heavily he always left an incentive factor in it so that the more a man produced from professional fees the more he took home. He also realized that people go through different phases of satisfaction in medicine. The fine young clinical investigator may find that later on in life he really gains more satisfaction from patient care than he does from the laboratory. A young man who is a superlative clinician and teacher may lose the excitement of teaching later in life and be an ineffective teacher while still maintaining great clinical expertise. Stead recognized that the private diagnostic clinic provided an opportunity for what he called "lateral movement" within the Department of Medicine. In essence, if an investigator or a good teacher found that he was gaining more and more satisfaction from the practice of clinical medicine he could easily be shifted into the PDC area. There he would not only gain his own personal satisfactions but he would continue the reputation of the institution for good clinical care and provide an even broader financial base for Stead to obtain venture capital. Thus, one of the primary arms of Stead's department was the private diagnostic clinic with its ability to generate unfettered dollars for him to use. I say *him* advisedly because these funds were totally at Stead's discretion. There was no research committee to allocate funds; there was no senior advisory committee to tell him how to invest the funds; it was a simple benign dictatorship.

When Stead arrived from Atlanta he not only recognized the potential of the PDC to generate funds for his purposes but he also recognized the great need to install a strong research program. Combining the dollars generated from the PDC, plus his unique ability to ferret out and raise funds from the federal government, he rapidly built a very strong research arm within the department. Just as he recognized that motivation was important in generating funds from the PDC, he also recognized that if his research people were put in a position of receiving financial rewards from seeing patients they would gradually, over the course of age, be tempted to forgo their research responsibilities. He therefore elected to salary these members of the faculty. Any income generated by their efforts in the patient care area went directly to Stead's coffers which further enhanced his venture capital account.

He never tried to keep in total balance salaries between those working primarily in the PDC and those who were working in research laboratories. His defense of this was that "time is money". If you wanted free time to pursue the things that interested you in the laboratory it might well cost you some money in terms of what you could normally generate from a clinical practice. On the other hand, the pressures of clinical practice were such that, if you were to generate your salary, there would not be a great deal of time to pursue a laboratory project. Thus he told the clinicians that they had no complaint about not having enough time to do what they wanted to do because if they wanted to create the time they could stop generating more income for themselves; he told his research arm that they could not complain about not receiving salaries equal to some of his clinicians because they had the free time to do what they wanted and were not encumbered by the unpredictable demands of a clinical practice.

For those who had worked in the department a significant amount of time, his concept of "lateral movement" defused the issue, because if a man who had been productive in the laboratory decided he wanted to generate more income and leave the laboratory there was a place for him in the clinical arena where he could generate more income. On the other hand, as occasionally happened, a clinician who found that his basic interests lay more toward the laboratory could tailor his schedule to the point where his income was curtailed and his free time was increased.

While this offered the potential and danger of generating two kinds of faculty, the system did not evolve in that direction, although there was a tendency toward it. All members of the department were expected to teach and, regardless of whether they were in the laboratory or in the private diagnostic clinic, they took their turns with various teaching and administrative responsibilities.

Stead The Educator

Although Stead strove throughout his career to instill quantification into medicine and to make it more of a science, he readily recognized that basically it is a pragmatic science at best. One of the keystones to his approach to the teaching and the practice of medicine was to be certain of what was truly known and not known, not only about a disease but also about a particular feature of the patient's history or physical examination. Unless he was reasonably certain of the facts he refused to arrive at a conclusion from an isolated clinical event. Nor would he allow his house officers to do so. This rigid demand for separation between "facts" and inference permeated his ward rounds and his analysis of complex research data. This simple but consistent intellectual demand allowed him to not only come down on the right side of a clinical judgment more often than not but it also made him an awesome reviewer of every scientific paper that came out of the diverse subspecialty laboratories of his department. It also made him uniquely compatible with the burgeoning computer age and made him very comfortable with the role of a leader of a major data analysis system which he took on as an administrative responsibility after he left the chairmanship of the department.

He, like Osler, felt that the central focus of teaching medicine was the patient. Every patient, no matter how mundane the complaint, was an interesting patient to him. Woe to the house officer who mentioned to Stead on the way to the bedside that this particular patient was not particularly interesting. The subsequently chagrined house officer would spend an hour or more at that bedside while Stead elicited a series of interesting observations about the patient's medical and personal life, all of this being interspersed with a series of piercing questions which the house officer neither had thought of nor was able to answer.

Rounding with Stead was much like playing tennis against a veteran player who barely seemed to move from position but had his house officers running all over the court frantically trying to retrieve adroitly placed drop shots. He might spend five minutes discussing a patient with classical pneumococcal pneumonia because his house officers had spent half the night in the library reviewing the literature on the latest advances in the treatment of and the pathogenesis of the disease. He knew they had learned the facts and there was no need to teach something already learned. On the other hand, he might well spend an hour-and-a-half at the bedside of a psychoneurotic middle-aged lady who had a host of medical complaints which could not be explained and an even larger number of personal problems that the house officer had never even elicited. This approach not only motivated his house officers to learn as much as they possibly could about disease and people but it also instilled in his house officers a concept of human charity which patterned their lives in the practice of medicine. He was a stickler for details when they concerned a vital decision in clinical medicine. He did not hesitate to have the junior resident draw pictures of the eyegrounds of multiple patients if the resident had indicated during teaching rounds that he did not have a detailed knowledge of a hypertensive patient's fundi.

Stead designed his career around teaching, whether it was teaching medical students, house officers, fellows or his young aggressive research oriented faculty. In order to implement his teaching philosophy, he recognized the need for a rigid system of teaching and the need for the frequent active input of the chairman. He was a believer in the trite adage that "when the cat is away the mouse will play". Therefore he was seldom away long enough for anybody to really know that he had left the institution. He rounded on Osler Ward three days a week, usually 11 months a year. He also had a physical diagnosis group of five or six second-year students who were just beginning their adventure in medicine. This heavy rounding schedule and exposure to all levels of learners in his department produced an all-pervading feeling that Stead was always around the corner and that at any point in time you might be called upon to explain your actions. This generated a level of compulsion in terms of providing medical care that was handed from generation to generation of house officers and students.

As another means of maintaining a vigorous teaching program, he insisted on a system of ward rounds in which the student presented the patient, the intern answered all those questions that the student couldn't, and finally when the intern "ran out of gas" the resident answered the questions the intern couldn't. He never believed there was any hierarchy of knowledge on rounds and was ever ready to listen to the student who seemed to know more about the patient or a complex biochemical abnormality than the resident, if the student clearly was the one with the pertinent information.

While Stead was a traditionalist in the sense of applying the above principles to medical education, he also was an innovator in medical education. He had long believed that the senior year in medical school should be the golden year, in which the student had enough basic science and clinical knowledge as well as reasonably unfettered time to incorporate these two areas into the fabric of his clinical practice. At some point in time, however, he began to realize that this was not how most medical students were using their senior year. This led him, along with others at Duke, to begin to revise their thinking about how to distribute time in the curriculum. At a lunch table conversation with some basic science chairmen the issue of the possibility of revising the curriculum came up. From this lunch table conversation evolved a new Duke curriculum which had a core basic science course in the first year followed by injection of the students into the ward teaching system in the second year, to be followed by a return to the basic sciences in the third year and eventually a return to clinical services in the fourth year.

This possibility had been germinating in Stead's mind because he recognized that much of the relevance of basic science was lost on the student until he had been exposed to pertinent questions in clinical medicine. Yet, in the old-fashioned curriculum with the first two years consisting of basic science and the last two years clinical science, there was no way to go back and recapture those areas of basic science which the third- or fourth-year student now knew were very pertinent. While the idea may have germinated it really took the addition of a new generation of young basic science chairmen at Duke to make the plan feasible. Traditionally the basic science departments had jealously guarded their two years with the student and Stead initially thought there would be no unbending of this position. However, I think much to his surprise, he found a group of basic science chairmen who were enthusiastic about this approach, since they felt that when they had the students return to them in the third year they would be dealing with an even more highly motivated group of students who might not only learn a great deal of more basic science but even be more inclined to join basic science research programs. Thus the new Duke curriculum was launched with enthusiasm from both basic science and clinical departments.

Another innovation in medical education stemmed from his belief that medicine was basically a practical science and that the principles of the care of the sick could be taught to people with average intelligence and superior motivation. He did not believe that a vigorous, highly structured premedical education background was needed to train people to take care of many medical problems. As a good researcher he launched his hypothesis with a pilot project that probably started with Thelma Ingles, who was a professor of nursing and very interested in patient care. Stead set aside an hour a day with Thelma to discuss and review the medical aspects of a particular patient that Thelma had become interested in while she was directing her student nurses on a ward. Thelma was an extremely talented woman in her own right and an apt student. Gradually over the course of the years she really became an extremely knowledgeable person about areas of medicine which usually were reserved for physicians.

Having shown to his own satisfaction that it didn't take a medical school or premedical background to develop this sort of knowledge in a motivated person, he recognized that the experiment ought to be extended to involve people who had shown some aptitude for medicine but who really had not had nearly the background that Thelma Ingles had had in nursing.

Because of his interest and also because of the needs of various patient-care oriented laboratories in the Department of Medicine, he began to actively encourage the recruitment of military corpsmen to come to the medical center to work in laboratories to see how they could be melded into the system of patient care. It became obvious that these people were extremely motivated and could rapidly become sophisticated in well-delineated areas of patient care. Having demonstrated this, Stead launched what has been perhaps one of the most unique projects in medicine, the physician's assistant program. This was pioneered at Duke under his initial guardianship. The successful development of the physician's assistant program was a logical extension of his fundamental concept that medicine was a practical science and that there was no hierarchy of knowledge so long as one learned to define what he did know and what he did not know.

Although Stead recognized that he was considered an outstanding medical educator, he would be the first to admit there was one area where he really made little impact in medical education; that was postgraduate medical education for the physician who had left the medical center. It is interesting to note that, although he was basically unsuccessful in generating a strong postgraduate medical program during his tenure as chairman, he turned his shoulder to the wheel after his retirement as chairman and has been instrumental in setting up a unique postgraduate training program involving Cabarrus Hospital in Concord, North Carolina. This model is being expanded to include a series of other hospitals and has been extremely helpful in orienting the Department of Medicine toward more participation in other publicly funded programs, such as the Area Health Education Centers (AHEC).

Stead And His Housestaff

Stead had a unique relationship and lasting effect on anyone who joined his housestaff. In many ways it might be characterized as a stern father-son relationship. He was admired because of his keen intellect and his ability to isolate the critical issues, whether they be clinical or administrative. He was also feared because he was quick to point out in no uncertain terms where he thought mistakes had been made. His constant presence in the medical center left every house officer with the sensation that Stead knew everything there was to know about him. Stead was bright enough to know that only an occasional indication that he knew what was going on was enough to indicate to the entire housestaff that he knew everything. This was obviously not the case, but Stead never let anyone think otherwise. This ever-present sensation bred a level of discipline within his housestaff which went on from year to year. He remained aloof in many ways from his housestaff during their first year or two in his program but, as he began to know them better as junior residents and they began to recognize that the demands he placed upon them were not that difficult to meet if one really cared about medicine, the relationship became warmer. For the house officer who had spent two or more years at Duke, Stead became vitally interested in his career and made every effort to open doors and seek support for his future training, whether it be in clinical medicine or in the laboratory.

When the roster of old housestaffs is reviewed and names from the past are recognized now as leaders in their field, one is tempted to think that Stead's housestaff was hand-picked and recruited from the finest institutions across the country in a selection process that would guarantee the success of his housestaff. Certainly during the early years this was far from true. In the late 40's and early 50's Stead's program was just getting off the ground at Duke and Duke was entering its first great growth phase since its foundation in the late 20's. There were catch-as-catch-can years in terms of housestaff recruitment and the intership slots were sometimes barely filled by the matching program. It is a tribute to the strength of the program Stead installed that some of the brightest lights in medicine today who were members of the early housestaffs came to Duke almost by chance and were not the hand-picked leaders of their medical school classes.

Stead believed that for the young house officer there was only one place and one way to learn medicine and that was to be in the hospital. He clearly stated that he didn't think a boy was likely to learn medicine at home asleep and that for the first several years of his medical training he ought to be totally immersed in the care of sick people. Early in his years at Duke, I doubt that he was particularly enamoured of the idea of having a house officer married since this would be a distracting influence. As a matter of fact, one of his house officers enjoys telling the story of how Stead was kind enough to give him two days off to get married rather than the one day that he had merited on the basis of the usual housestaff schedule.

Stead's firm belief that medicine could be learned only amongst the sick led to the development and persistence of the so-called five nights out of seven schedule which became famous, or infamous depending upon whether you were in or out of the program. In essence, while you were on the inpatient service, which for the first 12 years meant about 10 months out of the year, you spent five nights out of seven sleeping in the hospital and you didn't go home for supper or sleep. The usual rotation was that the intern or junior resident went home on Wednesday night and either Saturday or Sunday afternoon and evening. The majority of those who worked under that system griped mildly to moderately during their tenure, recognized its great merit, and then proudly trumpeted their trials or tribulations for the rest of their lives.

The great virtue of this system was that it provided adequate time to learn and to pick what one wanted to learn from a variety of activities in the hospital. There was no great pressure to rush home for supper since no one was going home for supper. This meant that during the day the house officer attended conferences he chose and many times accompanied his patients to procedures in specialty areas. Since the house officer was going to be in the hospital all night anyway, an afternoon admission that didn't require immediate medical attention could easily be "worked up" in the evening. Furthermore, since most of the housestaff were in the hospital the majority of the time, it meant less night work and more sleep for everyone.

It obviously brought a closeness and camaraderie among the housestaff since basically it was like returning to dormitory living for the vast majority of the week. Many a bull session in either the Baker House living area of Duke Hospital or the Durham VA Hospital house officer quarters provided more medical education and more direction to careers than any type of systematized learning program would. It was traditional for the housestaff to gather in the dining room for late supper at 10 o'clock. At that time it was almost inevitable that various patients and their problems were discussed and collective thoughts, opinions and recommendations were passed back and forth across the late supper table to the advantage of the entire housestaff.

To say that this system was met with universal acclaim would certainly be erroneous, particularly among the wives of house officers. Housestaff training under the five nights out of seven system was a testing ground, not only for house officers but also for young marriages. While some marriages may have foundered under these circumstances, the vast majority of them did not. In retrospect I think in many ways this initial exposure to the demands of medicine for a young marriage may have been far more educational to a couple than was ever realized. Many times, newly married wives were forced, for the first time, to recognize the commitment that their husbands had made to the practice of medicine. Many times, husband and wife had to learn to cope with the sacrifices and make a marriage work in a way which would recognize them and accommodate a series of com- promises within the boundaries of the practice of good medicine.

While the schedule was long it was almost universally rewarding to the house officer. Wives learned how to adapt themselves to living without their husbands a good portion of the time. There was less loneliness than might be expected, since it was a Duke tradition for the wives with their children to join their husband for dinner in the hospital dining room several nights a week. This made the Duke Hospital dining room look like a nursery on many occasions, but it also led to firm and lasting relationships between couples that met each other under these rigorous circumstances.

As times changed and the majority of housestaff arrived married, Stead recognized the importance of helping the wives to accommodate to their husbands' profession. During my tenure as chief resident he recruited my wife to form the Medical Housestaff Wives Club which was an instant success and is an even more active organization now when husbands are home more often.

In the early 1960's, Stead recognized that the five nights out of seven schedule no longer was in tune with the rest of medical housestaff programs. Furthermore, he realized that the old system served as an impediment for recruiting top-drawer students who could go to equally prestigious programs which advertised less awesome work schedules. The system was modified to allow the house officer to go home to his family when his work was completed, but much of the discipline generated by the original system pervades the present program.

Stead had a different philosophy about each rung on his housestaff ladder from intern through junior resident, senior resident and chief resident. Stead believed that there had to be one year in a boy's training where he had to develop efficiency and learn what was important to do rapidly and almost reflexly. This was the internship year. His philosophy was that during medical school the intern had been given a whole host of tools to take care of sick people. But he would never be an effective physician unless he learned to pick and choose these tools appropriately and use them so rapidly and efficiently that he could see a large number of patients and handle a large number of problems. He felt the only way to teach this efficiency was to be certain that the intern was so busy that he had to make some choices about what was going to be done and what was not going to be done. Stead readily recognized that in the process of making these decisions the intern would make mistakes but, unless the intern had to make a choice, he would never learn what was right and what was wrong about his decision. It was once aptly stated by one of Stead's lieutenants that "if the intern has time to go to the library there is something wrong with the program".

The intern who had been trained in medical school to retire to the library and the textbooks to find out exactly what he should know and do about a disease initially felt insecure in the system. It wasn't until he graduated to higher levels of the housestaff program that he realized that all along there had been a whole host of people around him who were there to provide him with information and to prevent him from making disastrous errors. The attending staff whose laboratories and offices were right in Duke Hospital were always available for discussions about patient problems. They frequently were wandering the wards in the evening checking patients they had studied and thus presented a ready opportunity for an unsure intern to obtain an informal consultation.

This system was not overly taxing to most interns; it was a once-in-a-lifetime growth experience for a smaller number, and a very unhappy time for an occasional intern. Stead never worried at length about the complaints of the interns unless he perceived that an individual's complaint was a cry for help. He did not expect his interns to become enamoured of the system and he did not expect instant loyalty from his interns. He took the position that the relationship between a new intern and the department was somewhat like a blind date: neither party knew each other beforehand, neither party quite knew what to expect from each other, and neither party should be angry with each other if the relationship didn't become a lasting one. On the other hand, he expected and received total loyalty from his residents. They knew the system, they had chosen to remain a part of it, and they were expected to make it work.

The bulwark of the housestaff system was really the junior resident. He had been through a vigorous internship, he had seen a large number of sick patients and he had gained the confidence and the efficiency which the internship had been designed to provide. He was basically the manager of the ward and his responsibility was to be certain that the patients were well taken care of and that his students and interns were learning a large amount of medicine. While the junior resident had this responsibility it was still considered an intern's service and the intern was the only one allowed to write orders on the chart. This seemingly contradictory system of responsibility without "authority" made many a junior resident exasperated early in his tour of duty. It dovetailed beautifully, however, with what Stead expected out of the junior resident. He recognized that unless his junior residents were mature enough to learn how to motivate and direct people under them, they would never become effective leaders in providing medical care. He also believed firmly in the hierarchy of knowledge and, if a junior resident with cogent reasons could not persuade an intern to take a particular course of action, then the resident had either insufficient knowledge or the intern insufficient understanding. In these rare cases the attending physician assigned to the ward was occasionally consulted but it seldom was necessary. The resident also had to learn how to get the best from the nursing staff. When an occasional conflict developed between the resident and a head nurse, Stead did not hesitate to point out that it was easier to recruit another resident than it was to recruit another veteran head nurse.

The senior assistant resident was a consultant as he rotated through the various subspecialty areas and had arrived in Nirvana because he had to be in the hospital only one night out of three; and he could come by, leave erudite notes and not be on the firing line worrying about where that next sick patient was going to come from and what time of the night he was going to arrive.

The chief resident was basically the chief executive officer for the day-to-day operation of the medical service, both on the private and the public service. He had a unique opportunity to get to know Stead because he sat with Stead and the residents from the private service at morning report from 8 to 8:30 every morning of the year except Sundays. A solid year of sitting with Stead, listening to his philosophy at morning report, left a lasting impression on all his chief residents. The chief resident was expected to know where the patient problems were, recognize house officers who were in trouble, shepherd through the various students who were taking junior medicine, placate an attending staff which occasionally was frustrated by seeming inadequacies of a house officer and, perhaps above all else, bring to Stead's attention any problems which the resident felt needed urgent attention.

The wise resident also learned that he didn't bring all the problems that he had to the attention of Stead. Stead's solutions were often quick and likely to create more problems for the chief resident than he originally had, so that one of the learning processes of the chief residency was to be certain that the potential solutions that Stead might offer would not bring more troubles for him. Thus, in many ways the chief resident was a buffer between some of his more recalcitrant housestaff and Stead. Stead dealt with his chief residents on an almost peer plane although the chief resident always knew who was boss. He obviously treated each chief resident differently and encouraged some to pursue more clinical pursuits if this was their area of weakness and others to pursue more intellectual avenues if they had already proven themselves outstanding clinicians.

There were several unique features of Stead's program which serve to demonstrate how differently he looked at the education of his housestaff. There were three events which were probably unique in American medicine. They included Stead's morning report, Sunday School, and "psychotherapy for the chief resident". Stead's morning report was held every day of the week except Sunday with the chief resident and the two residents from the private service. Stead set aside a half-hour each day to spend this time with the three house officers to talk about anything they wanted to talk about. The subject matter would range from medicine to politics or to even certain features of the entertainment world, including television and the movies. The ground rules for report were that this was the junior residents' time to discuss anything they wanted to with Stead and, if they didn't have anything to discuss, there would be no discussion, and by no discussion I mean silence—for 30 minutes if necessary. One of the agonizing roles of the chief resident was to be certain that not too many sessions of 30 minutes of silence occurred during a junior resident's four-week rotation. Needless to say, having a group of independent minded junior residents, there were occasions when the system was tested and the junior residents decided they would see if they could last 30 minutes without saying anything or without Stead saying anything. One of the chief resident's stock-in-trade was to have several provocative questions tucked in the back of his mind in case it looked like the group was headed for a period of prolonged silence but, despite such ingenuity, there were times when the bait wasn't taken and the silence returned.

A second institution or tradition which Stead enjoyed was Sunday School. Sunday School consisted of an hour-long presentation by a house officer on any medical topic of his interest. During the course of rotation through the year, each house officer gave one Sunday School lecture which was held at 9:30 Sunday morning and attended by most of the housestaff and a significant portion of the attending staff. Stead was in attendance at most of the meetings since he was in town so often. He was the first to probe piercingly the knowledge of the speaker. There is probably no Duke house officer who gave a Sunday School who can't, to this day, expound at length on the subject he discussed 15 or 20 years ago. In retrospect these sessions turned out to be extremely valuable, not only to the one presenting them but also to all those who attended, since over the course of several years of going to Sunday School weekly one became uniquely prepared to take his internal medicine boards. There was literally no subject of interest in medicine that wasn't covered during the course of several years as a house officer.

Finally, perhaps one of the most unique features of Stead's housestaff training program was the opportunity he gave to his chief residents to spend three hours a week with a clinical psychologist, Dr. Bingham Dai. When Stead was asked why in the world he would feel it necessary to send his chief residents, who were at least theoretically sane, to see a psychologist he replied, "I have never been certain that psychiatry had much to offer people who are insane but I think it makes a sane man more productive". Stead felt so strongly about this that he paid Dr. Dai's professional fee year after year to counsel the chief resident from Duke and from the VA Hospital. In actuality almost all the chief residents who did spend a year with Dr. Dai came away from the experience feeling that it was the best part of the entire chief residency experience.

It was not truly psychotherapy but more a session of character analysis. Although each resident's experience with Dr. Dai was obviously different, it did in general follow a pattern which even the chief residents recognized and joked about. There was a period of somewhere between three to six months where the resident was encouraged to talk about anything that happened to come to mind while Dr. Dai studiously maintained silence and scribbled rapidly on 5x8 cards. A description of dreams was particularly encouraged, for dream analysis was one of Dr. Dai's fortes. After this period Dr. Dai began to be more inquisitive and more directive. His questions began to expose the basic reasons and motivations behind day-to-day decisions made by the chief resident. The foibles, prejudices, compulsions, fears, etc. of each resident gradually came to the surface under Dr. Dai's gentle tilling. The resident left the experience knowing a great deal more about the reasons for his responses to stressful situations than he ever would have, if it were not for that experience. The sessions with Dr. Dai came at a very appropriate time, since the chief resident was operating under maximal self-imposed pressure trying to manage a complex, talented, and sometimes unruly housestaff in such a way that his demanding chairman would think the ship was still afloat. Under these perceived stresses it didn't take long for Dr. Dai to dissect any personality.

Stead The Administrator

Perhaps the real secret to Stead's ability as an administrator was that he understood people were different and that each person had his own motivational framework which was fruitless to tamper with. From this stemmed the concept of "lateral movement", or changing roles within the department which is discussed in relation to the private diagnostic clinic.

Stead's style of administrating was fascinating to watch. He encouraged, he threatened, he cajoled, he used all the techniques of a good administrator but at the very core of his administrative skill was his extreme efficiency in perceiving a problem and making a decision about a solution. Stead disciplined himself in such a way that he had more free time than anyone else in the department. Throughout the department he delegated not responsibility but opportunity. If a man was given an opportunity and seized it, it became his responsibility. If he didn't take the opportunity and, in turn, the responsibility, there was another man to take his place. In this way Stead freed himself of many of the petty administrative chores of running a department, and his younger men carried these along with their teaching and research responsibilities. He was always available to guide and advise and occasionally to veto, but he used to say, "Those young aggressive men don't bother me; I can get out of their way. It's the slow ones that I have trouble with because I have never learned how to make them move faster".

Stead not only used his lieutenants to free up his time but he also was extremely efficient in how he operated his department office. He and his loyal secretary, Mrs. Bess Cebe, between the two of them managed to operate a multimillion dollar operation without accountants, advisers, lawyers, etc. At 8:30 each morning, after morning report with his house officers, he would go to Mrs. Cebe's desk, open the right-hand upper drawer where there would usually be a small stack of papers which required his immediate decision. He would then sit on a small chair at Mrs. Cebe's side and write yes, no, not now, etc. Within a period of about 10 minutes he was ready for his day, roaming the laboratories and going to teaching rounds. He delegated the rest of his professional commitments to Bess to work out and his personal commitments he delegated to his wife, Evelyn. Between the two of them they were probably the most effective administrative aides in any department of medicine.

Stead was prone to delegate travel arrangements to whomever he was traveling with if his two best administrators, Bess Cebe and Evelyn Stead, were not along on the trip. He learned not to assign me such a task after I allowed both of us to miss a connecting flight in Washington while we enjoyed a leisurely beer. I was chagrined and implored him not to tell my wife about this bit of stupidity. His reply was, "On one condition: that you don't tell Bess or Evelyn".

All was not sweetness and light in a vigorously growing university such as Duke, and Stead was not a grandfatherly figure in his dealings with other chairmen, departments, the hospital, and the University. He had a strong department; he had a relatively financially independent department; he had a strong national power base; and he played the game for keeps. He won many battles and he lost a few. When he lost a contest he lived by the principle that if you are going to play the game you can't pick up your bat and ball and go home when you lose an inning. If he failed in a project once, he would retire without great rancor to try and figure out another way of getting the same thing done. He was tenacious in pursuing his goals but he was quick to recognize a lost cause and to cut his losses.

As a good administrator Stead really understood the value of the dollar. He brought the department reserve fund from a very small sum to a very large sum and in the process built a huge successful department, but he never paid a dime more than it would take to get a task done. He drove a hard bargain for hospital space and for beds, because he understood that this was the source of income for the department. He paid salaries which were respectable but they were by no means at the top rung of salaries for his young people coming along. He did this partly because he wanted to use every dollar available to build more within his department and also because he didn't want to keep his department static. The real desire to preserve as many dollars as possible for the department, plus the desire to have his people go out and make a name for themselves in other institutions was perfectly met by his salary policy. On the rare occasions when he was concerned about salary being a deciding factor in retaining a vital person in his operation, he took an unusual approach to the negotiations. He would call down the man who was being actively recruited by another institution just before the man was to leave for a visit to the recruiting institution. Stead would then tell the man being courted that he was going to tell him what his salary would be in the following year and that he did not want to get involved in salary negotiations with another institution. So, when the young man went to the other institution, he knew exactly what he would be making at Duke if he stayed. Stead then indicated that this was his only and final offer so, when the young man returned from his visit to the other institution, they could discuss other matters, but they were not going to discuss salary. I am sure this principle was occasionally bent for, although Stead was rigid as an administrator, he believed that "rules are made to be broken".

In many ways, Stead's financial operation in the Department of Medicine might be best described as the "rob Peter to pay Paul" principle. He had virtually total control of all the "taxed" dollars from the PDC and, indeed, much of the grant dollars that had been awarded to different sections of the department from outside agencies. He was committed to building a strong Department of Medicine and he was not averse to borrowing some funds from one grant to meet the needs of another project or another division of the department. He felt he was responsible to the total department and, if one of its divisions was rich and the other poor, he was inclined to be certain that the poorer division got the funds it needed to grow. For instance, for many years he had a large cardiovascular training grant in which there were stipends for research fellows. In addition to these stipends, the NIH offered special fellowships for projects which would be granted directly from the NIH. Stead encouraged all of his young people who were coming along in cardiology to apply for special grants and, if they were successful, the funds in the original training grant were "reprogrammed", all with the permission of the NIH, to other projects or other individuals who were in need. While this produced a mobile source of funds which were used to great advantage to the entire department, this approach did not meet with complete equanimity among the young cardiologists. When he was reproached for this, he said simply that he had never seen a good cardiology division in a bad department of medicine and that if the cardiologists wanted to have a good division of cardiology they needed a strong department of medicine. An overall review of his stewardship of funds certainly would indicate that this judgment was correct, but logic and success in his approach still didn't nake some of his decisions any less painful to the cardiologists.

Perhaps nothing more typifies Stead's insight into administration and his objectivity about people than the decisions he made about retiring from the chairmanship of the Department of Medicine. Stead retired at the age of 59 in 1967. He was at the height of his intellectual, academic and political powers and many could not fathom why he had done this. Most of those who did not know him did not realize that this decision to retire early had really come nine years before the implementation of the decision.

Despite the fact that he warned the powers that be in the medical center well ahead of time that he was going to resign from the chairmanship, the leadership of the medical center was unwilling to accept this initially. Indeed, a search committee which was eventually constituted to find his successor met to begin the screening process for a successor and finally adjourned with a vote to recruit him to be the next chairman of the Department of Medicine. Needless to say, Stead, who had made up his mind nine years previously to retire, indicated in no uncertain terms that the search committee had better find a new chairman because he was not going to be on the grounds when his predesignated resignation date arrived.

When I was chief resident he was in the active process of designing his resignation to be handed in nine years after that. He was quite open and free about discussing it and, indeed, it was the subject of more than several morning reports. His position was that he had never seen a department of medicine with a chairman above the age of 60 that had not deteriorated while the chairman reigned until his eventual retirement. His general observations had been reinforced by the fact that several chairmen whom he had admired a great deal had allowed themselves to stay in a position of power beyond the age of 60 and, just as he had noted in the past, their departments had deteriorated around them. He felt he had spent too much time and effort and had too much pride in his department to let this happen. He also recognized that, while he felt that way at the age of 50, he might not feel the same way at the age of 60. Thus, if he were going to truly resign, he would have to make his plans at the age of 50 in such a rigid fashion that there would be no impediment to his resignation 9 or 10 years hence. Stead also wished to insure the fact that the chairman who succeeded him would not have to carry his whole salary as a burden and thus limit the resources of the department in recruiting young people. With this in mind he saved during his tenure the money to pay the department's portion of his salary from age 60 to 70. The medical center agreed to increase the budget of the department for 10 years to cover their portion of the salary.

The new chairman had none of his money tied up in Stead. Stead believed that early retirement had many advantages to the school, but these advantages could be realized only by pre-retirement planning.

Stead: The Trainer of Medical Leaders

A perusal of the list of all the people who trained under Stead, and particularly his department and division heads who have gone on to other institutions, would lead one to believe that he was infallible in the choice of people for a specific position. This was not really the secret to his success in training medical leaders. The eventual blossoming of many medical leaders in his program stemmed from the fact that he brought to the department a system which had enough room and enough finances to allow young people to do their own thing. In essence, he took all the venture capital and all the other funds he could gather together and gave people an opportunity to succeed. He created the environment which consisted of free time, financial support, space and opportunity to grow and then sat back to see what happened. Many of those who chose to go in other directions than academic leadership used their several years that he sponsored to find that either they were not happy in an academic environment or they were not productive and thus they left to do other things.

His dealings with his chief residents were typical of this approach. Basically, the chief residency was considered by Stead to be a three-year tour. The first year was the chief residency year and then for the next two years the chief resident had the freedom to do whatever he wanted to do in the department while receiving a salary. At the end of two years, Stead sat down and compared the chief resident's growth with his peer group and they mutually agreed to continue on the faculty or he indicated that growth and productivity were not satisfactory to him and he would be glad to help the former chief resident achieve a position in another environment or institution.

Perhaps the best observation made about Stead's technique of training medical leaders was made by Dr. Jerome Harris who was then chairman of the Department of Pediatrics. He pointed out that it was uncanny how Stead had a large stock of young men who were given an opportunity to grow very early and, when new opportunities arose, he could always find someone among them to be a candidate for a new position.

In training his young faculty, Stead not only provided support but he was also ready to provide advice and direction if it was asked for—and sometimes when it wasn't asked for. He adapted his approach to each young faculty member in a different way depending on the skills of the individual. He tried to balance out their careers so that they were well versed, not only in their laboratory pursuits but also clinical medicine, so they could assume major responsibilities in large clinical departments. I have often heard the story that he inevitably asked Jim Wyngaarden how rounding on Long Ward was going, since Dr. Wyngaarden had been posted to nine consecutive months of rounds on the ward. He had been posted for that lengthy stay because he had been extremely productive as an investigator for several years at the NIH, and Stead wanted to be sure that his clinical skills were sharpened up for that day when Jim Wyngaarden would be running a department. On the other hand, Bill Deiss, who loved teaching clinical medicine, perhaps more than some of his laboratory pursuits, was always asked exactly how things were going in the laboratory, rather than how things were going in the teaching arena.

This individualization of approach to each of his young faculty provided an appropriate stimulus at an appropriate time. He was able to tolerate a host of almost eccentric aggressive young men as long as they were productive. Perhaps the quote that best characterizes his approach to this issue is, "You've got to be worth the trouble you create". He was quite willing to tolerate a great deal of trouble from productive people but he was intolerant of trouble from people who were not productive.

Although Stead appeared aloof and indeed threatening to his young faculty, he often had deep personal feelings about their growth and future. However, he never allowed these personal feelings to enter into major judgments about their careers in his department. If a man had been laboring at a problem for a long period of time and had not solved it or had not found an alternate problem that was solvable, Stead did not carry him on eternally, but sat down frankly with him and told him he was not productive enough to remain in his department. These decisions were undoubtedly hard for him but he made them on more than one occasion.

Understanding Stead

The first interview with Stead, whether as a house officer, young faculty member, or member of a visiting funding committee, often bordered on utter confusion. Stead seldom approached an interviewer or project without having thought at some length about the subject at hand. This thought process may have traveled over many different avenues of approach to the problem and incorporated many analogies. When he sat down to the interview, he was inclined on occasion to incorporate all his previous different approaches to solving a problem, but he was also inclined to omit some of the vital logical and chronological ingredients that went into his discussion. If you had lived with the idea and heard it several times from him and watched him manipulate ideas and political solutions, you could sit in on the interview and understand exactly why he was saying what he was saying. But if it was your first exposure to the problem or concept, the discussion could be utterly confusing. The young house officer who left Stead's office and said to himself, "I am not sure what he said", was really not that different from many others who were dealing on a much higher level of policy making. Part of this initial confusion stemmed, as I have indicated, from the fact that Stead had thought about the problem from many angles and was incorporating bits and pieces of the various resources leading to a solution. However, some of the confusion stemmed from the fact that he really used people as sounding boards to hear their objections, to see their responses to proposals, and to judge the acceptance of an idea so that he could further refine his own thinking about the problem. Eventually, once he had locked in place a combination of his own thoughts plus objections and refinements from others to whom he had talked, he would present the most lucid and compelling argument for or against a project. But, if you were caught in the in-between stages of the problem-solving process, it seemed almost like an idea game when nothing seemed to fit and no sentences were made.

Years of Growth: A Reprise

As I review this manuscript, I recognize all the errors of omission and commission an author can be guilty of. Perhaps the greatest is the failure to document Stead's growth as a man. He came to Duke as a brilliant, aggressive, sometimes abrasive young leader in medicine. In his early years these qualities brought great rewards to himself and to his department, but they also brought conflict and on occasion unhappiness to his staff and, I am sure, to himself. As the years passed, some of the rigidity which was his stock in trade gave way to tolerance of diversity which eventually became his strongest attribute as a teacher and an administrator.

His ability to continue to learn from life and people eventually led him to understand that not all men marched to the same drummer he incessantly heard. He recognized that some men placed higher values on some of the softer elements in life than he did. He not only became more tolerant of those attitudes but also used them to further motivate his men. He understood that man did not live by intellectual pursuits alone but gained strength from family and personal relationships which were originally outside Stead's disciplined intellectual bounds. As his interest broadened to his beloved lake house, which he literally built by hand, he began to realize that medical men, no matter how dedicated, had to have other pursuits that refreshed them and prepared them to face again the responsibility of providing good medical care every minute of every day.

Twenty-Six Years In Office

BESS M. CEBE

My 26 years of working for Dr. Stead have placed me in an enviable position. He has taught me, from 1951, as surely as he has taught the medical student, intern, resident, fellow, and upper staff. My advantage lies in not having had to leave at the end of the year, or after graduation, or when I'm offered a professorship elsewhere!

We started out in M-122, an area which also housed in its environs John Hickam and, down the hall, Jack Myers. Frank Engel was in the Bell Bldg. There were perhaps five small research grants in the Department, but each was vital, loved and protected. John and Jack were the right-hand men and alternated responsibility for the Department when Dr. Stead was away.

In about 1954, we moved to the first floor of Baker House, where Neurology now is. We were the first occupants of that newly-vacated nurses' residence. Soon thereafter, John and Jack moved to offices in Baker House basement (space now occupied by clinical cardiology).

Next we moved around the corner in Baker House—where the present Department of Medicine offices are. These were fine offices and, when the Medical PDC men asked me to persuade Dr. Stead to dress up his office with carpeting, new furniture, etc., he said he'd go along with the carpeting and drapery but only if my office was equally equipped. And so it was. He remained adamant about no new desk, saying that the one he'd used since 1947 had served him quite well and he saw no reason to replace it.

During my first week of working for Dr. Stead, he let me know the order of priority for his time: first, medical students; second, house staff; third, fellows; fourth, senior staff. He stayed more-than-busy all the time. With rare exception, he put himself on the teaching rounds schedule all year long, three mornings a week. He heard morning report at 8:00 A.M. six days a week. For many years, he read all manuscripts going out from the Department. He made a point of dropping in on division chiefs, labs, wards, etc., I suppose to (1) keep in touch with everything going on and (2) let people know that he was watching. He had a large hand in the Medical

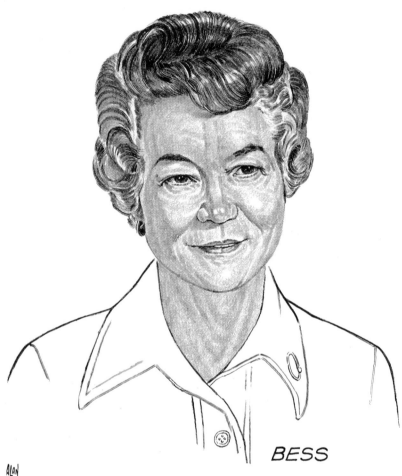

BESS

ALAN
MAVER

Private Diagnostic Clinic expansion, in moving the Outpatient Clinic from its small space to its present location, and in making application for, and getting, funds for the Diagnostic and Treatment buildings (1 & 2) and the Gerontology Building. He pushed hard for air conditioning on the wards, and got it. He had a large hand in the building and staffing of the VA Hospital in 1952. He ran Hypertensive Clinic one afternoon a week all alone for many years, and I was glad when Jack Wallace and Caulie Gunnells came along to help him. He taught a Physical Diagnosis section each year.

If you think he was busy then, here's what he is doing now: ward rounds thrice weekly for at least six months of the year, three afternoons weekly at the Methodist Home as attending physician and medical director, editor of *CIRCULATION*, considerable faculty and student guidance, inauguration and implementation of the computer textbook, and anything else that comes his way and needs doing.

As the years moved on and more space was needed, he solved the problem by having a portion of his office walled off for, first, Harry McPherson, second, Dick Portwood, and third, Jim Mau. His view was that my office was the one needing to stay the bigger one since "that's where all the work is done, and more people come in to see you than me."

When the D&T-2 bulding was in blueprint stage, plans were for us to move there and Dr. Stead asked me to sketch out possible use of the space. Because of the plumbing arrangement, one of us would have to be opposite the men's room. I sketched out the space, giving him of course the better section of the area. He said, "No, that won't do. You've been opposite the men's room all these years—it's my turn now." As things worked out, we didn't move to the new building. He believed other folk needed the space more than he did.

Like everyone, he had bad days along with the good. A bad day was easy to spot by 7:55 A.M. So, if a man was on the calendar that day and I knew he was coming to ask a favor or a blessing of Dr. Stead, I would rearrange the appointment and hope for a better day next time.

One could go on and on. On a Saturday morning in August 1967, he moved out of 121 Baker House to make room for Dr. Wyndaarden. I cried a little bit.

After about 16 months, which he spent away from Duke so as to cause as little interference as possible to Dr. Wyngaarden, we ended up in 281 Baker House.

1951–67 were hard years, but I wouldn't trade them for anything. He taught me how to grow up, how to separate the wheat from the chaff, how to manage problems and people, how to thrive on long hours and hard work, and how to be glad I did. [1977]

• 16 •

The Profit in Losing a Nickel*

GEORGE J. ELLIS, III, M.D.

When some of the residents were asked last summer what difference it made to have been exposed to Dr. Stead for just a few months, many answers were forthcoming. It was pointed out that on rounds he didn't teach or emphasize what a good intern or what a good resident might have. No one came away with a part list of "the six most common causes" or the "best" therapeutic program. Each student and house officer who worked with him on Osler Ward learned something different. Usually, each one learned what he needed most at the time to handle a difficult problem.

The one thing on which all house officers could agree that they learned from Dr. Stead was the meaning of a nickel bet. Nickel bets have been Dr. Stead's stock-in-trade since his intern days in Boston. They have become the cornerstone of medical education at Duke. These nickel bets were made during discussions of clinical problems that usually took place after leaving the bedside of the patient. The bet was not a frivolous gamble on the patient's fate. Instead, the nickel bet served three functions: first, it stimulated a meeting of the minds by defining differences of opinion; secondly, it stimulated data gathering in support of the arguments; lastly, it provided a time limit for settling the question.

Believe me, Dr. Stead's nickel stuck to the blackboard was a great stimulus towards answering clearly defined questions. It was not surprising that the loser of a nickel gained more than the winner. After all, he invested more energy in trying to save his nickel, and in the process he learned something he didn't know before.

In appreciation for this guidance in effective and precise learning and for the fun that we have shared as Osler physicians, the house staff presents to Dr. Stead a plaque bearing a great central buffalo nickel rendered in buffalo hide. One nickel was placed around the periphery of the rawhide nickel for

*Ann. Int. Med. **69**: 990, 1968

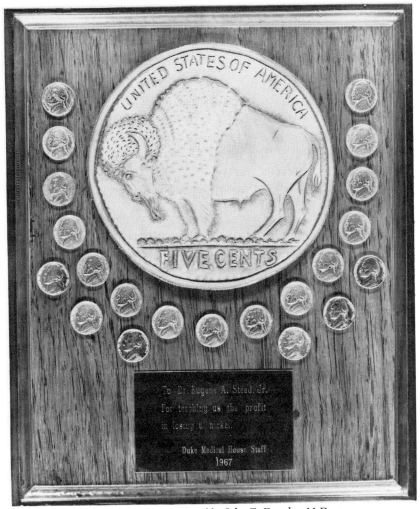

Designed and produced by John E. Douglas, M.D.

each of Dr. Stead's years as chief at Duke. The inscription on the plaque reads:

To Dr. Eugene A. Stead, Jr.
For teaching us the profit
in losing a nickel
Duke Medical House Staff
1967

17

To Yellowstone With A Forty-Eight Year Old:
Being Raised By Eugene Stead

WILLIAM W. STEAD, M.D.,*

Eugene Stead is known as an outstanding doctor, scientist and teacher. As his son, I was amazingly unaware of his professional achievements until recent years. I know him as a father, a role which he has handled with characteristic flexibility and imagination.

Eugene Stead is the man who carved a toy boat out of a 2x4 and made a concrete pond in the backyard. You could sit on his knee to hear the Perils of Pauline, each story ending in a precipitous drop to the floor. He went camping with the Boy Scouts and slept on the stump that was on his side of the tent. He built a rowboat, bought a 2½ horsepower motor, and took a day off to take an 18-mile boat ride. He used his leisure time to build the family a house on a lake, and he built it himself.

Growing up with Eugene Stead was not always cheerful. He did not believe in sparing the rod to spoil the child. When I was nine, he took the family West. We ate later than I would have liked and my attitude was repaid with a spanking as an appetizer before almost every dinner. He has often wanted to write a book about going to Yellowstone with a nine-year old, and thus the title of this section. His terse verbal truths were even more potent than spanking. Our family had the usual sibling rivalry, and it was in that context that I first heard that "the world is not fair" and that "life is hard".

My first recollection of my father in the hospital comes from a day I went to meet him after work. He ran down the halls of Baker House with me, yelling "Indians! Indians". The main impact his profession had on me was the times it took him away from home. I had a simple system for judging

*Associate in Medicine (Nephrology), Duke.

chief residents. The bad ones had morning report on Sunday. The good ones didn't and we could spend Saturday night at the lake.

My adolescence must have been a difficult time for my father. I had points of view that made sense to me at the time, but differed from his. He didn't argue; he said, "You'll understand when you grow up". That was like red to a bull, because I thought I was grown up and I thought I understood. In retrospect he was right more often than I like to admit.

Now that I am able to support myself, he has done what must be the hardest thing for a parent to do: he has let me live my own life. That doesn't stop him from giving advice. When I started my clinical rotations in medical school he took me for a walk to the Chapel. This represented the family equivalent of a housestaff walk in the Duke Gardens. His message was simple: no one will remember whether you know the differential diagnosis. They will only remember if you made their day easier and more exciting.

I have worked with my father in a variety of roles. He was my rounding man on Long Ward when I was an intern, and I have covered for him at the Methodist Home in recent years. I will probably forget most of those encounters, but I will not forget a night when I was a second-year medical student on 6A and he made guest attending rounds. It was his only appearance at the VA that summer, and the chief resident and all the ward residents were in attendance. I presented a patient with possible scleroderma. My father examined the patient while I was presenting. When he tried to take off the patient's slippers to examine his feet, the patient winced. (His feet were blistered.) I said, "Dr. Stead, don't do that". This had no effect, so I said, "Daddy, don't!" He stopped and nobody laughed.

Granted, Eugene Stead is an excellent physician, but he is a better father. I will also consider myself a "Stead man". [1977]

18

On Following In Gene Stead's Footsteps

JAMES B. WYNGAARDEN, M.D.*

Dr. Stead was the main reason for my choosing to come to Duke in 1956. I knew him only by reputation. He had been an original and creative cardiovascular scientist. He had built an extraordinary Department of Medicine at Emory. He had continued an outstanding record of building in a decade at Duke. But mostly those who had been associated with him spoke of his exceptional talents as a clinician, teacher, and stimulator of young people. He could get students, house officers, fellows and young faculty to reach heights they did not know they could reach.

When I visited Duke, the people I observed seemed to be having an exciting and interesting time. They worked incredibly hard and had fun doing it. These qualities appealed to me, so I joined his team.

Gene put great stress on producing people, bringing out their best talents, and preventing narrowness of development by involving them in all activities of the Department. In his professional career he produced over 30 department chairmen, numerous division chiefs, and hundreds of caring and thinking doctors.

Gene had observed that not all bright young leaders retained their enthusiasm and sharpness throughout a lifetime. He saw other departments peak and then atrophy under leaders who stayed too long. He insisted on retiring from the chairmanship by age 60, at the height of his powers. No one could persuade him to change his mind.

When in 1967 I was invited to return to Duke to succeed Gene as chairman of the Department of Medicine, my congratulations were mixed with condolences. Could anyone in fact function as chairman with Gene in the Department? These doubters did not know Gene. He took a year's leave of absence and lived in New York. On returning he developed a new

*Professor and Chairman, Department of Medicine, Duke.

career in the field of medical information in the application of the computer to medicine. He said "no" to most requests to serve on committees both within and without the Department of Medicine. He continued his first love, ward teaching, making attending rounds on Osler Ward 11 months of the year as he had for so long, later reducing this to six months per year. Thus his influence among students and house staff continued.

I have gone to Gene for advice many times in the past 10 years. He is unfailingly attentive, quite willing to express an opinion. But it is usually followed with a comment such as, "It is easy to give advice when you do not have responsibility. You have to weigh my ideas against many other problems in the Department, and make up your own mind."

Gene has come to see me on a few occasions, to discuss a problem in the Department that is on his mind. These occasions have been rare. A few times he has offered unsolicited advice, which from my own experience I know is likely to contain wisdom, worth heeding. But the beautiful part of our relationship has been that Gene has never come back a second time on the same subject, has never asked, "What did you do with that suggestion I made, the advice I gave you last month?"

I grew to admire Gene greatly when he was my chief. He set an example of administrative and academic leadership that would be hard for anyone to match. But having given up the reins, and with an appreciation for the problems of the chairman, he has been supportive, understanding, and helpful, a rich and valuable resource for me as for so many others in the school. [1977]

Appendix I

List of House Staff: Emory, 1942–47; Duke, 1947–67

EMORY HOUSE STAFF, 1942–47

1942-43
John B. Hickam,
   chief resident
Walter H. Cargill
Arthur B. Codington
J. Frank Harris
Julian C. Lentz
Edward S. Miller
Harry J. Price
James V. Warren

1943-44
Edward S. Miller,
   chief resident
Guy H. Adams
Thomas Armour
Gordon Barrow
Philip Bondy
Charles E. Brown
Charles D. Burge
Eugene Calloway
Walter H. Cargill
Arthur B. Codington
Tom Cook
Goodloe Erwin
Milton Freedman
Nathaniel Glover
J. Frank Harris
Bernard C. Holland
William S. Hooten
Fred Kern
Julian C. Lentz
Harry J. Price
William L. Paullin

Fincher C. Powell
Richard C. Rodgers
William W. Stead
John F. Stegeman
Harry H. Wagenheim

1944-45
J. Frank Harris,
   chief resident
Sayge H. Anthony
Gordon Barrow
Curtis Benton
Richard E. Boger
Charles E. Brown
Charles D. Burge
Curran S. Easley
William B. Fackler
Richard E. Felder
William N. Fitzpatrick
Glenville Giddings
Nathaniel Glover
William A. Hodges
Bernard C. Holland
George H. Holsenbeck
Henry S. Jordan
Fincher C. Powell
Peritz Scheinberg
William W. Stead
A. Calhoun Witham

1945-46
Charles Huguley,
   chief resident
Sayge H. Anthony

Curtis Benton
Richard E. Boger
Curran S. Easley
Richard E. Felder
William N. Fizpatrick
Glenville Giddings
William A. Hodges
Henry S. Jordan
William R. Kay
Rudolph Marshall
James F. Schieve
A. Calhoun Witham

1946-47
David F. James,
   chief resident
Ivan L. Bennett
Philip K. Bondy
H. Eugene Brown
Walter H. Cargill
Arthur B. Codington
Bernard L. Hallman
Thomas B. Haltom
Ralph A. Huie
Willoughby Lathem
Julian C. Lentz
Chester W. Morse
J. Spalding Schroder
Hyman Stillerman
William M. Straight
Henry F. Warden
John C. Withington

DUKE HOUSE STAFF, 1947–67

1947-48
Samuel P. Martin,
  chief resident
George C. Adams
Woodrow Batten
Frank Bone
Robert Broome
John R. Burgess
Walter B. Burwell
Walter Coker
Nathaniel Ewell
Paul Fillmore
Priscilla Foote
Robert Hall
Bernard C. Holland
H. W. Jayne
Ulfar Jonsson
Herbert King
William A. Lambeth
Willoughby Lathem
William E. Leeper
Myron D. Mattison
Rudolph McCullough
Theo H. Mees
William T. Parrott
Charles H. Peete
Robert Pinck
Hugh B. Praytor
William W. Pryor
Peritz Scheinberg
Eugene Taylor
Frederick A. Thompson
Benjamin Vatz
Robert W. Willett

1948-49
Bernard C. Holland,
  chief resident
Albert M. Attyah
Wilmer C. Betts
Gus Casten
Paul Fillmore
William Fitzpatrick
William J. Fleming
John Geibel

Carlton M. Harris
William Hodges
J. William Hollingsworth
Benjamin F. Huntley
Ulfar Jonsson
John Logue
William S. Lynn
Alan Ory
William W. Pryor
Charles Rast
Harold St. John
James F. Schieve
Marvin Silver
Arthur R. Summerlin
W. Jape Taylor
James Teaubeaut
Carl Voyles

1949-50
James F. Schieve,
  chief resident
Donald C. Carter
Gus Casten
Thomas E. Fitz
Jules Hirsch
Robert Hollett
J. William Hollingsworth
Benjamin F. Huntley
Ramon Lange
Harry T. McPherson
John Muller
Barbara Newborg
James F. Nickel
Alan Ory
Joseph Parker
Sam Phillips
Charles Rast
Jack G. Robbins
Hugh Sealy
Herbert O. Sieker
W. Jape Taylor
Eugene Towbin
Charles A. VanArsdall
Carl Voyles
Robert W. Willett

1950-51
Grace P. Kerby,
  chief resident
Roy A. Agner
Caroline Becker
Ivan L. Bennett
Lachlan Campbell
Wilma Canada
Gus Casten
Leighton Cluff
Thomas E. Fitz
Ben Friedman
Thomas Gorsuch
Ladd W. Hamrick
Reginald Henry
Murray Hunter
Carl Jaeger
Ramon Lange
William S. Lynn
Henry D. McIntosh
Harry T. McPherson
Robert L. McWhorter
Theo H. Mees
John Muller
Richard Murphy
Barbara Newborg
William W. Pryor
Lloyd H. Ramsey
Fabian Robinson
Ernest E. Schnoor
James L. Scott
Eugene J. Towbin
John M. Wallace
Charles D. Williams

1951-52
J. William Hollingsworth,
  chief resident
Roy A. Agner
Mary C. Becker
Med S. Brown
Donald D. Carter
C. Hilmon Castle
Howard Cox
Clifton Davenport

Elizabeth B. Decker
George A. Edwards
Arnold Fieldman
Thomas E. Fitz
Stephen R. Fromm
Tom L. Gorsuch
Ladd W. Hamrick
Murray B. Hunter
Robert Kibler
Ruth Kimmelstiel
Francis P. King
Thomas E. Langley
Herbert Lourie
William S. Lynn
Susan R. McFadyen
Barbara Newborg
Clark Reed
Gerald P. Rodnan
Robert Shimm
L. Myrl Spivey
Eugene J. Towbin
Millard W. Wester

1952-53
Gerald P. Rodnan,
   chief resident
Caroline Becker
Morton D. Bogdonoff
Robert Burch
Needham B. Carter
Thomas Cocky
Phin Cohen
Howard Cox
Clifton Davenport
Elizabeth Decker
E. Harvey Estes
Paul Fillmore
Thomas E. Fitz
Ben Friedman
Norman H. Garrett
William L. Gleason
H. LeRoy Izlar
Elizabeth Jackson
Carl Jaeger
Henry Johnson
Ruth Kimmelstiel
David Kipnis
William Lacy
Thomas Langley

Leonard Lister
Herbert Lourie
Fairfax Montague
John Morledge
Ernest B. Page
George R. Parkerson
Ellison C. Pierce
Clark Reed
Oscar Reinmuth
Hugh Sealy
Thomas Sharp
Charles VanArsdall
George Welch
Millard Wester
E. Jefferson White
Tiffany Williams
John W. Wilson

1953-54
Harry T. McPherson,
   chief resident
Daniel Donovan,
   chief resident
Raymond C. Appen
William G. Aycock
John Ayers
Robert Ayerst
James M. Bacos
John A. Barrett
Melvin Berlin
Stuart Bondurant
Needham B. Carter
Jerome E. Cohn
John T. Eagan
Paul Fillmore,
   chief resident 7/1-9/1
John F. Flanagan
R. Denis Giblin
William L. Gleason
Gerald S. Gordon
Wallace W. Harvey
William K. Helms
H. LeRoy Izlar
Tomas Jonasson
James C. Jones
George A. Kelser
David M. Kipnis
Amos Lieberman
Leonard Lister

John D. Lord
Robert L. McWhorter
Myron Melamed
Glenn Mortimore
H. Victor Murdaugh
George R. Parkerson
Ellison C. Pierce
Lawrence W. Pollard
Paul W. Seavey
Herbert O. Sieker
Delford L. Stickel
William L. Sutton
Eldora Terrell
Thomas E. Terrell
Charles VanArsdall
Tom A. Vestal
Rhett Walker
Donald E. Warren
Robert B. Welch
Robert W. Willett
John W. Wilson
Janet E. Wolter
Alexander H. Woods

1954–55
Morton D. Bogdonoff,
   chief resident
Henry D. McIntosh,
   chief resident
Gerald L. Alexander
William G. Aycock
John Ayers
James M. Bacos
John A. Barrett
Stuart Bondurant
C. Edward Buckley
James B. Clement
C. David Cooper
Robert H. Cress
Lamar Crevasse
Paul Didisheim
Bruce Draper
Herbert T. Dukes
George F. Elsasser
Andrew P. Ferry
Walter R. Gaylor
Gerald S. Gordon
Thomas L. Gorsuch
Fred W. Graham
Joae Graham

Sidney Grossberg
Wallace W. Harvey
William K. Helms
Wilmer C. Hewitt
Benjamin T. Jackson
Walter Lusk
A. Donald Merritt
Suydam Osterhout
Ernest B. Page
Henry E. Payson
Lillian Pothier
Robert Proper
Clark Reed
Roscoe R. Robinson
Donald Rucknagel
Farrokh Saidi
Wayne H. Schultz
Madison S. Spach
Eldora Terrell
Thomas E. Terrell
Thomas B. Thames
Dewey R. Tickle
John V. Verner
Tom A. Vestal
Rhett Walker
Donald E. Warren
Arnold M. Weissler
Roy A. Wiggins
Alexander Woods

1955-56
Suydam Osterhout,
chief resident
Alexander Woods,
chief resident
Gerald L. Alexander
John Ayers
John A. Barrett
David J. Becker
Norman H. Bell
Paul C. Bennett
Richard I. Birchfield
Herbert A. Burke
Gerald A. Bryant
Barton Carl
Joseph J. Combs
Robert H. Cress
Arthur K. David
George F. Elsasser

C. Richard Gill
John R. Gill
Thomas W. Gore
Thomas E. Hair
Joe B. Hall
Gordon H. Ira
Henry C. Johnson
C. Conrad Johnston
Herbert Kaplan
Robert F. Klein
Martin E. Liebling
Ben W. McCall
Charles Markham
Richard Marshall
H. Victor Murdaugh
Robert K. Myles
Robert G. Peeler
Clark Reed
Roscoe R. Robinson
Joseph C. Ross
Donald Rucknagel
Donald E. Saunders
Robert H. Saxton
Paul Seavey
William Shapiro
Palmer F. Shelburne
W. Kyle Smith
L. Myrl Spivey
Sheldon Steiner
Saul Strauss
Andrew S. Tegeris
James R. Warbasse
James O. Wynn

1956-57
A. Donald Merritt,
chief resident
H. Victor Murdaugh,
chief resident
John A. Barrett
Norman Bell
Tommy A. Bruce
Gerald Bryant
Joseph J. Combs
Marion Crenshaw
Lamar Crevasse
Arthur David
Noble David
Raymond Doyle

Laurie Dozier
David A. Drachman
John Eagan
Walter L. Floyd
Marshall Franklin
Samuel J. Friedberg
Leonard Garren
John R. Gill
Kenneth Gough
Joseph Grayzel
Joseph C. Greenfield
Herbert Horowitz
Herbert Kaplan
William C. Kappes
Alexander Kisch
Lewis Lefkowitz
John Lord
Walter Lusk
Leo Lutwak
George Magruder
W. Ed McGough
Michael C. McNalley
D. Edmond Miller
Robert Myles
Robert A. Nebesar
Edward E. Owen
Robert Peeler
Wilbur C. Pickett
Abdul N. Rahman
Joseph C. Ross
Jay P. Sanford
David Schottenfeld
Joseph Shands
C. Norman Shealy
Eng Meng Tan
Harold R. Silberman
Sheldon Steiner
Samuel P. Tillman
John V. Verner
James Warbasse
Robert E. Whalen
J. Earle White
James O. Wynn

1957-58
John V. Verner,
chief resident
Roscoe R. Robinson,
chief resident

Edward E. Anderson
James M. Bacos
John A. Barrett
Vincent H. Bono
Irwin A. Brody
Jack T. Collins
Thomas M. Constantine
James B. Creighton
Noble J. David
Raymond T. Doyle
Laurie Dozier
John Eagan
Thomas K. Earley
T. David Elder
John S. Evans
Charles W. Fairfax
John Flanagan
Samuel J. Friedberg
James W. Fulton
John A. Gergen
William Gleason
Joseph Grayzel
Joseph C. Greenfield
Sidney Grossberg
Thomas H. Harrison
Herbert S. Heineman
Herbert Horowitz
James C. Hurlburt
Herbert F. Johnson
James H. Johnson
O. William Jones
William R. Lewis
Michael McNalley
Francis L. Merritt
D. Edmond Miller
Samuel E. Myrick
Jack H. Oppenheimer
E. Eugene Owen
Henry T. Perkins
Wilbur Pickett
Richard T. Pillsbury
Albert H. Powell
Owen Reese
C. Vernon Sanders
Donald Saunders
William Shapiro
Julian S. Sleeper
Anthony Slewka
Angelo P. Spoto

Harold L. Stitt
Theofilos J. Tsagaris
T. Reeves Warm
Arnold M. Weissler
Robert E. Whalen
Ralph Zalusky

1958-59
Arnold M. Weissler,
  chief resident
John Flanagan,
  chief resident
Edward E. Anderson
Richard Bean
Kenneth R. Bingman
Norman Berry
Richard Birchfield
W. Kenneth Blaylock
Irwin Brody
C. Edward Buckley
C. Donald Christian
Allan I. Cohen
Jack Collins
Thomas Constantine
Eugene T. Davidson
Charles W. Fairfax
Robert A. Fischer
Edward Genton
Hillel J. Gitelman
Tom W. Gore
Joseph C. Greenfield
Lawrence Grolnick
Herbert S. Heineman
Patrick Henry
Rafael Hernandez
James C. Hurlburt
James H. Johnson
O. William Jones
Marvin Kahn
Robert F. Klein
John Laszlo
John E. Lee
Carl Lyle
James D. Mallory
John J. McPhaul
Henry C. Mellette
Charles E. Mengel
Francis L. Merritt
Charles Merwarth

Francis W. Michel
Jack Oppenheimer
E. Eugene Owen
William L. Page
Richard H. Parker
Henry T. Perkins
Virginia O. Porter
George H. Porter
Charles E. Rackley
Jerome C. Robinson
Wendell Rosse
Lewis Seager
Robert Shofer
Julian S. Sleeper
Anthony Slewka
Kambuzia Tabari
Howard K. Thompson
Jack W. Trigg
Donald H. Tucker
Andrew G. Wallace
Robert E. Whalen
Ralph Zalusky

1959-60
Robert E. Whalen,
  chief resident
William Gleason,
  chief resident
Robert S. Adelstein
Clyde V. Alexander
Richard L. Bean
Robert K. Blount
Rubin Bressler
C. Edward Buckley
Henry S. Campell
Arthur C. Chandler
Allan I. Cohen
Jack T. Collins
Thomas Constantine
Elmer A. Deiss
Fred M. Downey
Arthur L. Finn
Robert L. Fischer
Robert E. Gaddy
Ferd E. Garrison
John S. Gaskin
Hillel J. Gitelman
John G. Glover
Harvey E. Grode

J. Caulie Gunnells
William R. Harlan
Howard C. Harrison
Charles P. Hayes
Rafael R. Hernandez
James T. Higgins
Richard Hildebrandt
James C. Hurlburt
Gordon H. Ira
Marvin Kahn
Joseph Katz
Eugene R. Kelly
John A. Laszlo
Marvin Lewis
Martin E. Liebling
Myron B. Liptzin
Melvin Litch
Dean T. Mason
Frank M. Mauney
Ben S. McCall
John J. McPhaul
Charles Merwarth
D. Edmond Miller
Irwin B. Moore
Alan L. Morgenstern
James J. Morris
David S. Newcombe
Charles E. Rackley
Stewart R. Roberts
Lloyd H. Robertson
Wendell Rosse
Robert G. Sumner
Kambuzia Tabari
Andrew G. Wallace
Donald K. Wallace
Temple W. Williams

1960-61
Howard K. Thompson,
 chief resident
Martin E. Liebling,
 chief resident
Thomas A. Andreoli
Norman Bauman
John O. Binns
William Blackard
W. Kenneth Blaylock
Robert K. Blount
Henry S. Campell

Allan I. Cohen
Ronnie Cox
Franklin P. Dalton
Stuart H. Danovitch
John Gaskin
Robert H. Gibbs
Tom W. Gore
William R. Harlan
Charles Harris
George M. Henry
Brunildo A. Herrero
Gordon H. Ira
O. William Jones
Eugene R. Kelly
Robert F. Klein
William B. Kremer
John H. Lane
E. Joseph LeBauer
Bernard Levy
Marvin Lewis
Joseph W. Linhart
John A. Lowder
R. Wayne Mall
Walter B. Mayer
Richard V. McCloskey
Ernest P. McCutcheon
James A. McFarland
Michael E. McLeod
David K. Meriney
Charles E. Merwarth
D. Edmond Miller
Richard J. Mountjoy
Irwin Moore
John B. Nowlin
Richard A. Obenour
Robert Peeler
Edwin T. Preston
Charles C. Richardson
David K. Rubin
Jerome Ruskin
Harold Silberman
Kenneth Starling
Robert G. Sumner
Kambuzia Tabari
Joel R. Temple
Robert W. Thompson
Leif O. Torkelson
Lawrence C. Walker
Andrew G. Wallace

Donald K. Wallace
H. Lake Westfall
Charles I. Williamson

1961-62
Charles Mengel,
 chief resident
Harold Silberman,
 chief resident
Thomas A. Andreoli
Michael F. Ball
Norman Bauman
Victor S. Behar
W. Kenneth Blaylock
Neil C. Brown
Joseph K. Bush
Freddie Butler
Joseph Cohn
Joseph J. Combs
Marcus A. Conant
Victor S. Constantine
David Culton
T. David Elder
Thomas ElRamey
Glen Finlayson
William Fore
Jane Fiscus
W. Guy Fiscus
Robert Gaddy
Saul Genuth
Cyrus Guynn
Charles Harris
Thomas H. Harrison
G. Morrison Henry
Patrick H. Henry
Rafael Hernandez
David H. Holloway
Harry Huneycutt
Edmund Katibah
Ralph Klopper
William B. Kremer
Joseph W. Linhart
Bernard Levy
Michael E. McLeod
Irwin B. Moore
James J. Morris
John B. Nowlin
Richard A. Obenour
Robert H. Peter

John Petralli
James Powell
Albert Powell
William Ridgeway
Jerome Ruskin
Fred Schoonmaker
L. Wade Self
William S. Smith
Donald Stewart
Charles P. Summerall
Joel R. Temple
John A. Trant
Carl Trygstad
Donald H. Tucker
Robert Waldman
Donald K. Wallace
G. Doyne Williams
Robert L. Young
Ralph Zalusky

1962-63
T. David Elder,
 chief resident
J. Caulie Gunnells,
 chief resident
Michael F. Ball
William A. Baxley
Victor S. Behar
Henry M. Bowers
Richard I. Breuer
Robert S. Brice
William D. Burton
Joseph K. Bush
Richard P. Carson
Ronnie L. Cox
Joe B. Currin
David K. Dunn
Joseph C. Farmer
Arthur L. Finn
Emile L. Gebel
Hillel J. Gitelman
Cyrus H. Guynn
Charles W. Harris
Thomas Harrison
Martin A. Hatcher
David H. Holloway
Edward S. Horton
Harry Huneycutt
Noel C. Hunt

Danny B. Jones
Kenneth J. Kahn
Martin S. Knapp
Nicholas M. Kredich
Edgar H. Levin
Harold J. Lynch
Patrick A. McKee
Earl N. Metz
Donald S. Miller
Sidney E. Morrison
James W. Myers
William A. Nebel
Francis A. Neelon
Donald W. Paty
Robert H. Peter
Charles M. Porter
Thomas Pozefsky
Norman B. Ratliff
Stewart R. Roberts
Fred Schoonmaker
Samuel D. Spivack
Bruce P. Squires
Richard C. Stone
Robert G. Sumner
Dean R. Taylor
Barry R. Tharp
John M. Thompson
H. Leonard Turner
Gail R. Williams
Temple Williams
C. Ivey Williamson
Howard J. Zeft

1963-64
Andrew G. Wallace,
 chief resident
James J. Morris,
 chief resident
Raymond H. Alexander
Willis H. Bell
Bernard A. Bernstein
John P. Boineau
Richard I. Breuer
Joseph O. Broughton
Joseph K. Bush
William A. Carter
Charles T. Caskey
William S. Collins
Wesley A. Cook

Joe B. Currin
Anthony R. Dowell
Doyle Driver
Ray R. Durrett
G. Jay Ellis
William W. Fore
Sidney R. Fortney
Robert E. Gaddy
William M. Ginn
Sheldon Goldgeier
Harvey E. Grode
Lee S. Harris
Charles E. Harrison
H. Courtenay Harrison
Chester C. Haworth
Edward S. Horton
William M. Hull
Marvin Kahn
Julian Katz
Peter O. Kohler
Lester J. Krasnogor
Nicholas M. Kredich
Samuel J. Lathan
Charles M. Mansbach
Richard V. McCloskey
Huey G. McDaniel
J. Frederic Mushinski
James W. Myers
Bert W. O'Malley
Alexander G. Reeves
Jerome Ruskin
Haskel Schiff
Fred W. Schoonmaker
Richard K. Shadduck
John S. Simmonds
William T. Sparrow
Samuel D. Spivack
Richard C. Stone
Dean R. Taylor
Joel R. Temple
Barry T. Tharp
John M. Thompson
Bart L. Troy
Roger W. Turkington
John E. Watt
H. Lake Westfall
Alan C. Whitehouse
Noel W. Young
Howard J. Zeft

1964-65
Michael E. McLeod,
  chief resident
Fred W. Schoonmaker,
  chief resident
Robert S. Adelstein
Page A. Anderson
Thomas E. Andreoli
Crawford F. Barnett
Willis H. Bell
Bernard A. Bernstein
John G. Blount
Joseph O. Broughton
Gene A. Butcher
Charles T. Caskey
Fred R. Cobb
Stanley N. Cohen
Frank P. Dalton
John L. Dobson
Anthony R. Dowell
Marshall C. Dunaway
Ray R. Durrett
Carl Eisdorfer
Robert O. Friedel
Jack K. Goldman
Richard Gorenberg
Allan M. Greenberg
Clarence E. Grim
Harvey E. Grode
Jordan U. Gutterman
Frank T. Hannah
Lee S. Harris
H. Courtenay Harrison
Joe T. Hartzog
Paul W. Hathaway
Brunildo A. Herrero
David H. Holloway
Gilbert S. Hunn
Herbert E. Kann
John R. Karickhoff
Julian Katz
Lester J. Krasnogor
William B. Kremer
Joseph E. LeBauer
David W. Martin
Richard V. McCloskey
Patrick McKee
Robert C. Noble
Bert O'Malley

David F. Paulson
Carl S. Phipps
Samuel D. Ravenel
Carl J. Rubenstein
B. Winfred Ruffner
Jerome Ruskin
Stephen F. Schaal
Haskel Schiff
Philip T. Shiner
Spencer Shropshire
John S. Simmonds
Roger W. Turkington
Abe Walston
John E. Watt
H. Lake Westfall
Alan C. Whitehouse
Douglas P. Zipes

1965-66
Earl N. Metz,
  chief resident
Brunildo A. Herrero,
  chief resident
Michael J. Andriola
Tryggvi Asmundsson
Goeffrey H. Basson
Wiley R. Bland
John B. Blount
Joseph O. Broughton
Gene Butcher
Harry M. Carpenter
Thomas P. Clancy
Harvey J. Cohen
Ronnie L. Cox
Frank P. Dalton
Bruce W. Dixon
John E. Douglas
Marshall C. Dunaway
Ray R. Durrett
G. Jay Ellis
Fred Ginn
Robert Gilgor
Clarence E. Grim
Jordan U. Gutterman
Russell E. Harner
Lee S. Harris
David H. Holloway
Ronald J. Karpick
Richard I. Katz

Stewart E. Kohler
Kenneth R. Krauss
Stephen M. Kulvin
Charles M. Mansbach
Huey G. McDaniel
George Massing
David W. Martin
Robert C. Noble
James J. Nordlund
Thomas Pozefsky
Allan H. Pribble
Andrew R. Price
Charles P. Riley
Stephen G. Rostand
B. Winfred Ruffner
Edwin A. Rutsky
Stephen F. Schaal
Haskel Schiff
Robert J. Schwartzman
Philip T. Shiner
Kirkwood T. Shultz
Ralph Snyderman
Henry L. Stewart
George S. Strauss
Dean R. Taylor
Jack B. Taylor
Joel R. Temple
Barry Tharp
John M. Thompson
Galen S. Wagner
Abe Walston
John W. Weeks
Douglas P. Zipes

1966-67
Harry M. Carpenter,
  chief resident
Anthony R. Dowell,
  chief resident
Richard A. Appen
George R. Blumenschein
Ernest C. Borden
J. Kerry Bush
Gene A. Butcher
Fred R. Cobb
Harvey J. Cohen
Glenn R. Cunningham
Walter E. Davis
Harry K. Delcher

Vincent W. Dennis	Kenneth A. Krauss	Jesse E. Roberts
Mark L. Entman	Gerald Logue	Stephen G. Rostand
Barry W. Festoff	Leif A. Lohrbauer	Michael Rotman
Sidney R. Fortney	James L. Males	Marvin P. Rozear
Michael Freund	Douglas J. Miller	Edwin A. Rutsky
John T. Garbutt	James L. Nash	Jerome E. Rygorsky
Paul M. Gertman	Albert R. Newsome	Robert J. Schwartzman
James H. Gordon	Laurance B. Nilsen	George S. Scott
Timothy E. Guiney	James J. Nordlund	Jack B. Sewell
Elliott B. Hammett	Charles B. Norton	Kirkwood T. Shultz
Charles B. Herron	James G. Nuckolls	David L. Smith
Christie B. Hopkins	William H. Obenour	Peter D. Springberg
Ronald J. Karpick	Thomas Pozefsky	Ralph Snyderman
Richard I. Katz	Andrew R. Price	Karl D. Straub
George L. Kline	Kenneth E. Quickel	Galen S. Wagner
Stewart E. Kohler	Charles B. Riley	Kinsman E. Wright

Appendix II

List of Department Chairmen Trained by Stead

PAUL B. BEESON: Chairman, Medicine, Emory; to Chairman, Medicine, Yale; to Radcliffe Infirmary, England; to Seattle VA Hospital

IVAN L. BENNETT: Chairman, Pathology, Hopkins; to vice-president, New York University Medical School

KENNETH BLAYLOCK: Chairman, Dermatology, Virginia

MORTON D. BOGDONOFF: Chairman, Medicine, Abraham Lincoln School of Medicine; to Executive Associate Dean and Professor of Medicine, Cornell

STUART BONDURANT: Chairman, Medicine, Albany Medical College; to Dean, Albany Medical College

RUBIN BRESSLER: Chairman, Pharmacology, Arizona; to Chairman, Medicine, Arizona

C. HILMON CASTLE: Chairman, Family and Community Medicine, Utah

LEIGHTON CLUFF: Chairman, Medicine, Florida at Gainesville; to Robert Wood Johnson Foundation

WILLIAM P. DEISS: Chairman, Medicine, Texas at Galveston

RICHARD V. EBERT: Chairman, Medicine, Minnesota

E. HARVEY ESTES: Chairman, Community Health Sciences, Duke

ABNER GOLDEN: Chairman, Pathology, Kentucky

SIDNEY E. GROSSBERG: Chairman, Microbiology, Medical College of
   Wisconsin
JOHN B. HICKAM: Chairman, Medicine, Indiana
BERNARD C. HOLLAND: Chairman, Psychiatry, Emory
J. WILLIAM HOLLINGSWORTH: Chairman, Medicine, Kentucky
WALLACE R. JENSEN: Chairman, Medicine, George Washington; to
   Chairman, Medicine, Albany Medical College
DAVID KIPNIS: Chairman, Medicine, Washington University
WILLIAM H. KNISELY: Chairman, Institute of Biology & Medicine,
   Michigan State; to vice-chancellor for health affairs, Texas; to president,
   Medical University of South Carolina
PETER O. KOHLER: chairman, Medicine, Arkansas
JAMES LEONARD: chairman, Medicine, Pittsburgh
SAMUEL P. MARTIN: chairman, Medicine, Florida at Gainesville; to
   Wharton School of Finance, Pennsylvania
HENRY D. MCINTOSH: chairman, Medicine, Baylor
CHARLES E. MENGEL: chairman, Medicine, Missouri
A. DONALD MERRITT: chairman, Genetics, Indiana
H. VICTOR MURDAUGH: chairman, Medicine, South Carolina
JACK D. MYERS: chairman, Medicine, Pittsburgh; to University Professor,
   Pittsburgh
JOSEPH C. ROSS: chairman, Medicine, South Carolina
PERITZ SCHEINBERG: chairman, Neurology, Miami
THEODORE B. SCHWARTZ: chairman, Medicine, Rush-Presbyterian
JAMES V. WARREN: chairman, Medicine, Texas at Galveston; to chairman,
   Medicine, Ohio State
ARNOLD M. WEISSLER: chairman, Medicine, Wayne State
JAMES B. WYNGAARDEN: chairman, Medicine, Duke

Appendix III

Curriculum Vitae, E. A. Stead, Jr.

Birthplace and date: Atlanta; October 6, 1908
Education: B.S., 1928, Emory University
          M.D., 1932, Emory University
Experience: 1932–33: Intern, Medicine, Peter Bent Brigham Hospital
          1933–34: Research Fellow, Medicine, Harvard

1934–35: Intern, Surgery, Peter Bent Brigham Hospital

1935–36: Assistant resident, Medicine, Cincinnati General Hospital

1936–37: Resident, Medicine, Cincinnati General Hospital

1937–39: Assistant in Medicine, Harvard and Boston City Hospital

1939–41: Instructor in Medicine, Peter Bent Brigham Hospital

1941–42: Associate in Medicine, Harvard

1942–46: Professor of Medicine and Chairman, Department of Medicine, Emory University

1945–46: Dean, Emory University School of Medicine

1947–67: Professor of Medicine and Chairman, Department of Medicine, Duke University

1967: Professor of Medicine, Duke University'

Other Activities

Past secretary and past president, Association of American Physicians

Past secretary and past president, American Society for Clinical Investigation

Master, American College of Physicians

Member, Association of University Cardiologists

Member, American Heart Association

Past member, Research Allocation Committee, American Heart Association

Past chairman, Ethics Committee, American Heart Association

Founding Member, National Academy of Sciences Institute of Medicine

Past member, Panel on Space Science and Technology [NASA] of the President's Science Advisory Committee

Member, American Medical Association

Past member, Council of the National Heart Institute

Past member, Council of the National Institute of Arthritis and Metabolic Diseases

Past consultant to National Heart Institute, Artificial Heart and Myocardial Infarction Program

Past member, Advisory Council, Life Insurance Medical Research Fund

Past director, Regenstrief Foundation for Research in Health Care

Editor, CIRCULATION, American Heart Association, 1973–78

Established training program for physician's assistants at Duke University, 1965

Honors and Awards

Phi Beta Kappa

Alpha Omega Alpha

Distinguished Professor, Duke University

Honorary Fellow, American College of Cardiology

Citation for Distinguished Service to Research, American Heart Association, 1959

The John M. Russell Award, Markle Foundation, 1968

Distinguished Teacher Award, American College of Physicians, 1969

The Robert H. Williams Award, Association of Professors of Medicine, 1970

James B. Herrick Award, American Heart Association, 1970

Abraham Flexner Award for Distinguished Service to Medical Education, Association of American Medical Colleges, 1970

Founder's Award, Southern Society for Clinical Investigation, 1973

Honorary degree: Doctor of Science, Emory University, 1968

Honorary degree: Doctor of Science, Yale University, 1971

Distinguished Teaching Award, Duke Medical Alumni Association, 1974

Georgia Heart Association, Symposium in Honor of Eugene Stead, 1976

Gold Heart Award, American Heart Association, 1976

Publications

1. Bryan AH, Evans WA, Fulton MN and ———. Diuresis following the administration of salyrgan. Arch. Int. Med. **55**: 735-744, 1935.

2. Gregersen MI, Gibson JJ and ———. Plasma volume determination with dyes: errors in colorimetry; use of the blue dye T-1824. Am. J. Physiol. **113**: No. 1, September 1935.

3. ——— and Kunkel P. A plethysmographic method for the quantitative measurement of the blood flow in the foot. J. Clin. Invest. **17**: 711, 1938.

4. Kunkel P and ———. Blood flow and vasomotor reactions in the foot in health, in arteriosclerosis, and in thrombo-angiitis obliterans. J. Clin. Invest. **17**: 715, 1938.

5. Kunkel P ——— and Weiss S. Blood flow and vasomotor reactions in the hand, forearm, foot and calf in response to physical and chemical stimuli. J. Clin. Invest. **18**: 225, 1939.

6. ——— and Kunkel P. Influence of the peripheral circulation in the upper extremity on the circulation time as measured by the sodium cyanide method. Am. J. Med. Sci. **198**: 49, 1939.

7. —— and Kunkel P. Mechanism of the arterial hypertension induced by paredrinol. J. Clin. Invest. **18**: 439, 1939.

8. —— and Kunkel, P. Factors influencing the auricular murmur and the intensity of the first heart sound. Am. Heart J. **18**: 261, 1939.

9. ——, Kunkel P and Weiss S. Effect of pitressin in circulatory collapse induced by sodium nitrite. J. Clin. Invest. **18**: 673, 1939.

10. —— and Weiss S. Effect of paredrinol on sodium nitrite collapse and on clinical shock. J. Clin. Invest. **18**: 679, 1939.

11. —— and Kunkel P. Nature of peripheral resistance in arterial hypertension. J. Clin. Invest. **19**: 25, 1940.

12. —— and Kunkel P. Absorption of sulphanilamide as an index of the blood flow in the intestine of man. Am. J. Med. Sci. **199**: 680, 1940.

13. Ebert RV and ——. The effect of the application of tourniquets on the hemodynamics of the circulation. J. Clin. Invest. **19**: 561, 1940.

14. —— and Ebert RV. The peripheral circulation in acute infectious diseases. Med. Clin. North America **24**: 1387, 1940.

15. ——. Changes in the circulation produced by poor postural adaptation. Bull. New England Med. Center **2**: 290, 1940.

16. Romano J, —— and Taylor ZE. Clinical and electroencephalographic changes produced by a sensitive carotid sinus of the cerebral type. New England J. Med. **223**: 708, 1940.

17. Ebert RV and ——. An error in measuring changes in plasma volume after exercise. Proc. Soc. Exper. Biol. & Med. **46**: 139, 1941.

18. —— and Ebert RV. Relationship of the plasma volume and the cell plasma ratio to the total red cell volume. Am. J. Physiol. **132**: 411, 1941.

19. —— and Ebert RV. The action of paredrinol after induction of hemorrhage and circulatory collapse. Am. J. Med. Sci. **201**: 396, 1941.

20. —— and Ebert RV. Postural hypotension; a disease of the sympathetic nervous system. Arch. Int. Med. **67**: 546, 1941.

21. Ebert RV and ——. Demonstration that in normal man no reserves of blood are mobilized by exercise, epinephrine and hemorrhage. Am. J. Med. Sci. **201**: 655, 1941.

22. Ebert RV and ——. Demonstration that the cell plasma ratio of blood contained in minute vessels is lower than that of venous blood J. Clin. Invest. **20**: 317, 1941.

23. ——. The treatment of circulatory collapse and shock. Am. J. Med. Sci. **201**: 775, 1941.

24. Ebert RV and ———. Circulatory failure in acute infections. J. Clin. Invest. **20**: 671, 1941.

25. Ebert RV, ——— and Gibson JG. Response of normal subjects to acute blood loss. Arch. Int. Med. **68**: 578, 1941.

26. Schales O, Ebert RV and ———. Capillary tube Kjeldahl method for determining protein content of 5 to 20 milligrams of Tussie fluid. Proc. Soc. Exper. Biol. & Med. **49**: 1, 1942.

27. ———and Ebert RV. Shock syndrome produced by failure of the heart. Arch. Int. Med. **69**: 369, 1942.

28. Ebert RV, ———, Warren JV and Watts WS. Plasma protein replacement after hemorrhage in dogs with and without shock. Am. J. Physiol. **136**: 299, 1942.

29. ———, Ebert RV, Romano J and Warren JV. Central autonomic paralysis. Arch. Neurol. Psychiat. **48**: 92, 1942.

30. Warren JV, Walter CW, Romano J and ———. Blood flow in the hand and forearm after paravertebral block of the sympathetic ganglia. Evidence against sympathetic vasodilator nerves in the extremities of man. J. Clin. Invest. **21**: 665, 1942.

31. Schales O, ——— and Warren JV. Nonspecific effect of certain kidney extracts in lowering blood pressure. Am. J. Med. Sci. **204**: 797, 1942.

32. Warren JV and ———. The effect of the accumulation of blood in the extremities on the venous pressure of normal subjects. Am. J. Med. Sci. **205**: 501, 1943.

33. Weiss S, ———, Warren JV and Bailey OT. Scleroderma heart disease. Arch. Int. Med. **71**: 749, 1943.

34. ——— and Warren JV. Clinical significance of hyperventilation: the role of hyperventilation in the production, diagnosis and treatment of certain anxiety symptoms. Am. J. Med. Sci. **206**: 183, 1943.

35. Warren JV, Merrill AJ and ———. The role of the extracellular fluid in the maintenance of a normal plasma volume. J. Clin. Invest. **22**: 635, 1943.

36. ———. The Pathologic Physiology of Generalized Circulatory Failure and of Cardiac Pain. In A Textbook of Medicine. Ed: Cecil, 6th ed., W. B. Saunders Co., Phila., 1943, pp. 1017-1030.

37. ———. Circulatory Collapse and Shock. In A Textbook of Medicine. Ed: Cecil, 6th ed., W. B. Saunders Co., Phila., 1943, pp. 1199-1202.

38. Warren JV and ———. Fluid dynamics in chronic congestive heart failure. Arch. Int. Med. **73**: 138, 1944.

39. —— and Warren JV. The effect of the injection of histamine into the brachial artery on the permeability of the capillaries of the forearm and hand. J. Clin. Invest. **23**: 279, 1944.

40. —— and Warren JV. The protein content of the extracellular fluid in normal subjects after venous congestion and in patients with cardiac failure, anoxemia and fever. J. Clin. Invest. **23**: 283, 1944.

41. —— and Warren JV. Care of the patient with chronic heart disease. Med. Clin. North America **28**: 381, 1944.

42. ——. Shock. Kentucky Med. J., May 1944.

43. Warren JV, ——, Merrill AJ and Brannon ES. Chemical, clinical and immunological studies on the products of human plasma fractionation. IX. The treatment of shock with concentrated human serum albumin: a preliminary report. J. Clin. Invest. **23**: 506, 1944.

44. Warren JV and ——. The protein content of edema fluid in patients with acute glomerulonephritis. Am. J. Med. Sci. **208**: 618, 1944.

45. Cooper FW, —— and Warren JV. The beneficial effect of intravenous infusions in acute pericardial tamponade. Ann. Surg. **120**: 822, 1944.

46. —— and Warren JV. Orientation to the mechanisms of clinical shock. Arch. Surg. **50**: 1, 1945.

47. ——, Warren JV, Merrill AJ and Brannon ES. The cardiac output in male subjects as measured by the technique of right atrial catheterization. J. Clin. Invest. **44**: 326, 1945.

48. Brannon ES, Merrill AJ, Warren JV and ——. The cardiac output in patients with chronic anemia as measured by the technique of right atrial catheterization. J. Clin. Invest. **44**: 332, 1945.

49. Warren JV, Brannon ES, —— and Merrill AJ. The effect of venesection and the pooling of blood in the extremities on the atrial pressure and cardiac output in normal subjects with observations on acute circulatory collapse in three instances. J. Clin. Invest. **44**: 337, 1945.

50. ——. Shock syndrome in internal medicine. Oxford Medicine **2**: 1 3, 1945.

51. Warren JV, —— and Brannon, ES. The cardiac output in man: a study of some of the errors in the method of right heart catheterization. Am. J. Physiol. **145**: 458, 1946.

52. Brannon ES, ——, Warren JV and Merrill AJ. Hemodynamics of acute hemorrhage in man. Am. Heart J. **31**: 407, 1946.

53. Merrill AJ, Warren JV, ——— and Brannon ES. The circulation in pene- trating wounds of the chest: a study by the methods of right heart cathe- terization. Am. Heart J. **31**: 413, 1946.

54. Warren JV, Brannon ES, ——— and Merrill AJ. Pericardial tamponade from stab wound of the heart and pericardial effusion of empyema: a study utilizing the method of right heart catheterization. Am. Heart J. **31**: 418, 1946.

55. ———, Brannon ES, Merrill AJ and Warren JV. Concentrated human albumin in the treatment of shock. Arch. Int. Med. **77**: 564, 1946.

56. ———, Hickam JB and Warren JV. Mechanism for changing the cardiac output in man. Trans. Asso. Am. Phys. **60**: 74, 1947.

57. ——— and Warren JV. Cardiac output in man. An analysis of the mecha- nisms varying the cardiac output based on recent clinical studies. Arch. Int. Med. **80**: 237, 1947.

58. ———. Fainting. In Signs and Symptoms. Ed: MacBryde. J. B. Lippincott, Phila., 1947, pp. 179-187.

59. ———. Relation of the cardiac output to the symptoms and signs of con- gestive heart failure. Modern Concepts of Cardiovasc. Dis. **16**: No. 12, 1947.

60. Warren JV, Brannon ES, Weens HS and ———. Effect of increasing the blood volume and right atrial pressure on the circulation of normal subjects by intravenous infusions. Am. J. Med. **4**: 192, 1948.

61. Scheinberg P, Dennis EW, Robertson RL and ———. The relation be- tween arterial pressure and blood flow in the foot. Am. Heart J. **35**: 409, 1948.

62. ———, Warren JV and Brannon ES. Cardiac output in congestive heart failure. Am. Heart J. **35**: 529, 1948.

63. ———, Warren JV and Brannon ES. Effect of lanatoside C on the circu- lation of patients with congestive heart failure. Arch. Int. Med. **81**: 282, 1948.

64. Scheinberg P and ———. The cerebral blood flow in male subjects as measured by the nitrous oxide technique. Normal values for blood flow, oxygen utilization, glucose utilization and peripheral resistance, with obser- vations on the effect of tilting and anxiety. J. Clin. Invest. **28**: 1163, 1949.

65. ———. Edema of heart failure. Bull. New York Acad. Med. **24**: 607, 1948.

66. ———. The role of the cardiac output in the mechanisms of congestive heart failure. Am. J. Med. **6**: 232, 1949.

67. ———. Circulatory factors in congestive heart failure. Trans. 3rd Conf.,, Josiah Macy, Jr. Foundation **178**, May 1949.

68. ———. Dietary and diuretic management of congestive failure. North Carolina Med. J. **2**: 54, 1950.

69. ———. Heart failure. Proc. 1st Natl. Conf. Cardiovascular Diseases. Am. Heart Asso., New York, pp. 157-160, 1950.

70. Scheinberg P, ———, Brannon ES and Warren JV. Correlative observations on cerebral metabolism and cardiac output in myxedema. J. Clin. Invest. **29**: 1139, 1950.

71. ———, Myers JD, Scheinberg P, Cargill WH, Hickam JB and Levitan BA. Studies of cardiac output and of blood flow and metabolism of splanchnic area, brain and kidney. Trans. Asso. Am. Phys. **63**: 241, 1950.

72. ———. Circulatory Collapse and Shock. In Textbook of Medicine. Ed: Cecil & Loeb. W. B. Saunders Co., Phila., 1951, pp. 1211-1214.

73. ———. Pathologic Physiology of Generalized Circulatory Failure. The Treatment of Congestive Heart Failure, Cardiac Dilatation and Hypertrophy. In Textbook of Medicine. Ed: Cecil & Loeb. W. B. Saunders Co., Phila., 1951, pp. 1051-1066.

74. ———. Renal factor in congestive heart failure. Circulation **3**: 294, 1951.

75. ———. Cerebral blood flow and metabolism. Am. J. Med. **9**: 425, 1950.

76. Murphy RJ and ———. Effects of exogenous and endogenous posterior pituitary antidiuretic hormone on water and electrolyte excretion. J. Clin. Invest. **30**: 1055, 1951.

77. ———. Edema and dyspnea of heart failure. Bull. New York Acad. Med. **28**: 159, 1952.

78. Holland BC and ———. Effect of vasopressin (pitressin)-induced water retention on sodium excretion. A. M. A. Arch. Int. Med. **88**: 571, 1951.

79. Bell DM and ———. Effects of epinephrine on the vessels of the calf. Observations on the period of initial vasodilatation. J. Appl. Physiol. **5**: 228, 1952.

80. ———. Fainting. Am. J. Med. **13**: 387, 1952.

81. ———. Presidential Address: Proc. 45th Annual Meeting, American Society for Clinical Investigation, May 1953. J. Clin. Invest. **32**: 548, 1953.

82. ———. Treatment of chronic and undiagnosed illnesses. GP **8**: 73, 1953.

83. ———. Peripheral Vascular Disease. In Textbook of Medicine. Ed: Cecil & Loeb. Blakiston, New York, 1954, pp. 1437-1448.

84. ⸺. General Considerations of Pain. **In** Principles of Internal Medicine. Ed: Harrison. McGraw-Hill, New York, 1954, pp. 17-20.

85. Holland BC and ⸺. Electrolyte excretion after single doses of ACTH, cortisone, desoxycorticosterone glucoside and motionless standing. J. Clin. Invest. **33**: 132, 1954.

86. ⸺. Circulatory Collapse and Shock. **In** Textbook of Medicine. Ed: Cecil & Loeb. W. B. Saunders Co., Phila., 9th ed., 1955, pp. 1261-1264.

87. ⸺. Diseases of the Cardiovascular System. **In** Textbook of Medicine. Ed: Cecil & Loeb. W. B. Saunders, Phila., 9th ed., 1955, pp. 1230-1246.

88. ⸺ and Hickam JB. Heart Failure. Disease-a-Month. Year Book Publishers, Inc., Chicago, 1955, pp. 3-32.

89. Burnum JF, Hickam JB and ⸺. Hyperventilation in postural hypotension. Circulation **10**: 362, 1954.

90. ⸺ and Warren JV. Controlling obesity with low fat cookery. Am. Acad. Gen. Pract. **15**: 98, 1957.

91. ⸺. Fainting (Syncope). **In** Signs and Symptoms. Ed: MacBryde. J. P. Lippincott, 3rd ed., 1957, pp. 665-678.

92. ⸺ and Wallace JM. Reactivity of small blood vessels. Trans. Asso. Am. Phys. **70**: 275, 1957.

93. Orgain ES and ⸺. Congestive heart failure. Circulation **16**: 291, 1957.

94. Wallace JM and ⸺. Spontaneous pressure elevations in small veins and effects of norepinephrine and cold. Circul. Res. **5**: 650, 1957.

95. ⸺. Congestive heart failure. Modern Medicine **26**: 164, 1958.

96. ⸺. Peripheral Vascular Disease. **In** Principles of Internal Medicine, McGraw-Hill, New York, 1958, pp. 1339-1348.

97. ⸺. Diseases of the Cardiovascular System. Circulatory Collapse and Shock. **In** Textbook of Medicine. Ed: Cecil & Loeb, 10th ed., W. B. Saunders, Phila., 1959, pp. 1172-1187 and 1199-1202.

98. Wallace JM and ⸺. Fall in pressure in radial artery during reactive hyperemia. Circul. Res. **7**: 876, 1959.

99. ⸺. Hyperventilation. Disease-a-Month, February 1960, pp. 5-31.

100. Wallace JM, Garcia H and ⸺. Arteriovenous differences of the norepinephrine-like material from normal plasma and infused norepinephrine. J. Clin. Invest. **40**: 1387, 1961.

101. Gorten R, Gunnells JC, Weissler AM and ———. Effects of atropine and isoproterenol on cardiac output, central venous pressure and mean transit time of indicators placed at three different sites in the venous system. Circul. Res. **9**: 979, 1961.

102. ———. Pain in the Extremities. In Principles of Internal Medicine. Ed: Harrison. McGraw-Hill, New York, 1962, pp. 56-60.

103. ——— and Kinney TD. Clinicopathologic Conferences, Duke University School of Medicine. So. Med. J. **55**: 410, 1962.

104. ———. Meaning of human behavior to the physician of tomorrow. Editorial. Arch. Int. Med. **110**: 409, 1962.

105. ———. Medical care: its social and organizational aspects. Postgraduate medical education in the hospital. New England J. Med. **269**: 240, 1963.

106. ———. The evolution of the medical university. J. Med. Educ. **39**: 368, 1964.

107. ——— and Greenfield JC. Pressures and pulses. Physiology for Physicians **2**: March 1964.

108. ——— and Greenfield JC. Pressures and pulses. Trans. Asso. Life Insurance Medical Directors of America **48**: 164, 1964.

109. ———. An internist looks at behavior. Billings Lecture. J. A. M. A. **195**: 157, 1966.

110. ———. Hyperbaric oxygenation. Editorial. Circulation 34: 361, 1966.

111. ———. Preparation for practice. Pharos of AOA **29**: 70, 1966.

112. ———. Challenge and opportunity. Editorial. Medical Times **94**: 370, 1966.

113. ———. Your National Library of Medicine. Editorial. Medical Times **94**: 507, 1966.

114. ———. The many facets of asbestosis. Editorial. Medical Times **94**: 633, 1966.

115. ———. Hypertension — highways and byways. Editorial. Medical Times **94**: 766, 1966.

116. ———. Looking at the heart. Editorial. Medical Times **94**: 884, 1966.

117. ———. Intern and residency training. Editorial. Medical Times **94**: 1001, 1966.

118. ———. Hyperbaria. Editorial. Medical Times **94**: 1128, 1966.

119. ———. On bacterial endocarditis. Editorial. Medical Times **94**: 1250, 1966.

120. ———. Reversible "madness". Editorial. Medical Times **94**: 1403, 1966.

121. ———. "Good will toward men". Editorial. Medical Times **94**: 1535, 1966.

122. ———. Current concepts. Training and use of paramedical personnel. New England J. Med. **277**: 800, 1967.

123. ———. Health manpower. Editorial. Medical Times **95**: 116, 1967.

124. ———. The lung. Editorial. Medical Times **95**: 235, 1967.

125. ———. Quality of medical care. Editorial. Medical Times **95**: 356, 1967.

126. ———. Traps and stratagems of diagnosis. Editorial. Medical Times **95**: 588, 1967.

127. ———. Thinking ward rounds. Editorial. Medical Times **95**: 706, 1967.

128. ———. Patients that recover. Editorial. Medical Times **95**: 802, 1967.

129. ———. The Duke plan for physician's assistants. Editorial. Medical Times, January 1967.

130. ———. Prevention of myocardial reinfarction. Editorial. Medical Times **95**: 899, 1967.

131. ———. Postural hypotension. Editorial. Medical Times **95**: 1120, 1967.

132. Cleland J, Aitken P, Bryson E, Hohman L, Jones T, Menefee E, Peete W and ———. The right to live and the right to die. Medical Times **95**: 1171, 1967.

133. ———. The rights of the foetus. Editorial. Medical Times **95**: 1226, 1967.

134. ———. The birth of a new educational venture — the association of schools of allied health professions. Editorial. Medical Times **96**: 99, 1968.

135. ———. The delivery of health care. Editorial. Medical Times **96**: 216, 1968.

136. ———. Educational programs and manpower. Bull. New York Acad. Med. **44**: 204, 1968.

137. ———. More knowledge about the renal factors influencing sodium excretion. Editorial. Medical Times **96**: 665, 1968.

138. ———. Myocardial infarction — the first 15 minutes. Editorial. Medical Times **96**: 665, 1968.

139. ———. Health and illness. Editorial. Medical Times **96**: 75 , 1968.

140. ———. A college-based physician's assistant program. Editorial. Medical Times **96**: 847, 1968.

141. ———. Cost conscious doctors. Editorial. Medical Times **96**: 947, 1968.

142. ———. The need for a machine processable medical data base. Editorial Medical Times **96**: 1154, 1968.

143. ———. Words make pictures. Editorial. Medical Times **96**: 1249, 1968.

144. ———. The limitations of teaching. Pharos of AOA **32**: 54, 1969.

145. ———. What we have learned about myocardial infarction from epidemiologic and dietary studies. Circulation **40**: IV-85, 1969.

146. ———. The role of the university in graduate training. J. Med. Educ. **44**: 739, 1969.

147. ———. The assets of a community hospital. Editorial. Medical Times **97**: 225, 1969.

148. ———. Picking other people's brains. Editorial. Medical Times **97**: 264, 1969.

149. ———. To manage or not to manage. Editorial. Medical Times **97**: 241, 1969.

150. ———. A National Academy of Medicine. Editorial. Medical Times **97**: 234, 1969.

151. ———. Space biology and medicine — an unmet challenge. Editorial. Medical Times **97**: 228, 1969.

152. ———. The physician's assistant -- job description and licensing. Editorial. Medical Times **97**: 246, 1969.

153. ———. Public assistance and society. Editorial. Medical Times **97**: 231, 1969.

154. ———. The white bear syndrome. Editorial. Medical Times **97**: 256, 1969.

155. ———. Why moon walking is simpler than social progress. Editorial. Medical Times **97**: 248, 1969.

156. ———. "Clinical trials" for proposed legislation? Editorial. Medical Times **97**: 187, 1969.

157. ———. Pain in the Extremities. **In** Harrison's Principles of Internal Medicine. Ed: Wintrobe. McGraw-Hill, New York, pp. 79-81, 1970.

158. ———. Vascular Disease of the Extremities. **In** Harrison's Principles of Internal Medicine. Ed: Wintrobe. McGraw-Hill, New York, pp. 1265-1274, 1970.

159. ———. Medical education and practice. Ann. Int. Med. **72**: 271, 1970.

160. ———. Congestive heart failure revisited. Editorial. Medical Times **98**: 200, 1970.

161. ———. Angina pectoris teaches. Editorial. Medical Times **98**: 201, 1970.

162. ———. "Origin of the Species". Editorial. Medical Times **98**: 223, 1970.

163. ———. Dialogue in California. Editorial. Medical Times **98**: 204, 1970.

164. ———. Universal service -- a necessity and an opportunity. Editorial. Medical Times **98**: 217, 1970.

165. ———. "If I become ill and unable to manage my own affairs ..." Editorial. Medical Times **98**: 191, 1970.

166. ———. Up the health staircase. Editorial. Medical Times **98**: 21 , 1970.

167. ———. Fainting (Syncope). **In** Signs and Symptoms. Ed: MacBryde. J. P. Lippincott, Philadelphia, pp. 712-721, 1970.

168. ———. A proposal for the creation of a compulsory national service corps. Arch. Int. Med. **127**: 89, 1971.

169. ———. Why moon walking is simpler than social progress. Pharos of AOA **34**: 3, 1971.

170. ———. Physicians -- past and future. Arch. Int. Med. **127**: 703, 1971.

171. ———. Use of physicians' assistants in the delivery of medical care. Ann. Rev. Med. **22**: 273, 1971.

172. ———, Editor: with CM Smythe, CG Gunn and MH Littlemeyer. Educational technology for medicine: roles for the Lister Hill Center. J. Med. Educ. **46**: 11-93, 1971.

173. ———. The way of the future. Presidential Address. Trans. Asso. Am. Phys. **85**: 1-5, 1972.

174. ———. Building a school. Am. J. Dis. Children **124**: 34 , 1972.

175. Rosati RA, Wallace AG and ———. The way of the future. Arch. Int. Med. 1 **1**: 285, 1973.

176. ———. Information and chronic illness. Editorial. J. Intn. Research Communications, November 1973.

177. Anlyan WG, Austen WG, Beck JC, Bradford WD, Brown RE, Cherkasky M, Elam LC, Kinney TD, London IM, Medearis DN, ——— and vander Kloot WG. The Future of Medical Education. Duke University Press, 1973. 192 pp.

178. ———. Chapter in Hippocrates Revisited. Ed: R. J. Bulger. Medcom Press, New York, 1973. 2 8 pp.

179. ———. Walter Kempner: a perspective. Arch. Int. Med. **133**: 755, 1974.